Contents

Contributors

Andrew H. Crenshaw, Jr., MD
Assistant Professor, Campbell Clinic of Orthopedic Surgery, University of Tennessee Center for Health Sciences, Memphis, Tennessee

Rodney Davis, MD
Division of Urology, Tulane University School of Medicine, New Orleans, Louisiana

Elise Hardy, MD
Division of Endocrinology, Diabetes and Metabolic Diseases, Jefferson Medical College of Thomas Jefferson University, Philadelphia, Pennsylvania

Diane M. Hershock, MD
Assistant Professor of Medicine, Hematology–Oncology Division, Department of Medicine, University of Pennsylvania Cancer Center, University of Pennsylvania Health System, Philadelphia, Pennsylvania

Ann Honebrink, MD
Assistant Professor, Department of Obstetrics and Gynecology, University of Pennsylvania Health System; Medical Director, Penn Health for Women, Philadelphia, Pennsylvania

Serge A. Jabbour, MD
Assistant Professor of Clinical Medicine, Division of Endocrinology, Diabetes, and Metabolic Diseases, Jefferson Medical College of Thomas Jefferson University, Philadelphia, Pennsylvania

Augustine S. Lee, MD
Senior Associate Consultant, Pulmonary and Critical Care Medicine, Mayo Clinic Jacksonville, Jacksonville, Florida

Richard Malamut, MD
Clinical Assistant Professor of Neurology, Drexel University College of Medicine, Philadelphia, Pennsylvania

Mary Gail Mercurio, MD
Assistant Professor of Dermatology, Strong Memorial Hospital, University of Rochester Medical Center, Rochester, New York

Joseph R. Pisegna, MD
Chief, Division of Gastroenterology and Hepatology, VA Greater Los Angeles Healthcare System, West Los Angeles Healthcare Center, Los Angeles, California; Associate Professor of Medicine, University of California, Los Angeles, California

Cynthia M. Tracy, MD, FACC
Associate Director, Division of Cardiology, Professor of Medicine, George Washington University Medical Center, Washington, DC

Preface

Lange Practice Tests: USMLE Step 1 was designed to be an up-to-date mirror of the Step 1 examination. The content and question types are designed around the current USMLE guidelines.

The questions are original and were produced by a faculty of clinicians who are both experts in their respective fields and physicians who are deeply involved with current teaching programs at their medical institutions. In this manner, you, the medical student, are assured of material that is both appropriate and accurate.

This guide will help you immensely in your studies for the USMLE Step 1 examination. Good luck on your exam!

Joel S. Goldberg
Philadelphia, Pennsylvania

Acknowledgments

I would like to extend my sincere appreciation to my editor, Ms. Catherine Johnson, for her assistance in the development of this project, along with the many staff members of McGraw-Hill who participated in this work.

I also wish to thank the physicians who participated in this project. They were able to find the time in their busy schedules to help in the creation of this work, which will benefit medical students across the United States.

Practice Test 1
Questions

DIRECTIONS (Questions 1 through 50): Each of the numbered items or incomplete statements in this section is followed by answers or by completions of the statement. Select the ONE lettered answer or completion that is BEST in each case.

1. A 72-year-old hypertensive man presents with acute onset of expressive aphasia and right hemiparesis affecting the face and arm more than the leg. Which of the following cerebral blood vessels is likely to be occluded?

   (A) left anterior cerebral artery
   (B) left middle cerebral artery
   (C) left posterior cerebral artery
   (D) right vertebral artery
   (E) basilar artery

2. A 71-year-old hypertensive woman presents with acute onset of Horner's syndrome, right face and left body sensory loss, dysphagia, dysarthria, and right limb dysmetria. Which of the following cerebral blood vessels is likely to be occluded?

   (A) left anterior cerebral artery
   (B) left middle cerebral artery
   (C) left posterior cerebral artery
   (D) right vertebral artery
   (E) basilar artery

3. A 64-year-old woman is admitted to the hospital with change in mental status. On exam, she has loss of the lateral third of her eyebrows. Which of the following does she most likely have?

   (A) adrenal insufficiency
   (B) pheochromocytoma
   (C) hypothyroidism
   (D) hyperparathyroidism
   (E) thyroid cancer

4. A 45-year-old woman presents with pretibial myxedema. Her laboratory studies will most likely reveal which of the following?

   (A) high thyroid-stimulating hormone (TSH) and low free thyroxine (T_4)
   (B) high TSH and high free T_4
   (C) low TSH and low free T_4
   (D) low TSH and high free T_4
   (E) normal TSH and normal free T_4

5. A 60-year-old postmenopausal woman sustains a hip fracture. Results of a bone density study are consistent with severe osteoporosis. Which of the following therapeutic agents does not inhibit osteoclastic activity in bone?

   (A) conjugated equine estrogen
   (B) 1,25-dihydroxyvitamin D [1,25(OH)2D]
   (C) calcitonin
   (D) alendronate
   (E) Miacalcin nasal spray

6. What is the most likely diagnosis in a 62-year-old man who has smoked cigarettes since the age of 15 and has a lesion on his lip?

   (A) basal cell carcinoma
   (B) squamous cell carcinoma
   (C) sarcoidosis
   (D) bite fibroma
   (E) melanoma

7. A 59-year-old woman presents to your office complaining of a 2-month history of early satiety and abdominal bloating. On pelvic exam you detect a 6-cm right adnexal mass and mild abdominal distention with a an air–fluid wave on abdominal exam. Subsequent pelvic ultrasound shows a complex right adnexal mass with a normal left adnexa and uterus as well as a moderate amount of ascites. Assuming that the patient's diagnosis is an ovarian malignancy, which of the following blood tests would you expect to be abnormal in this patient?

(A) alpha-fetoprotein (AFP)
(B) beta subunit of human chorionic gonadotropin (B-hCG)
(C) estradiol
(D) CA 125
(E) CEA

8. A 75-year-old man presents with a 6-month history of progressive difficulty ambulating. There is no history of trauma or leg pain. He has noticed that he has to lean against the wall as he walks, or he will lose his balance and fall. On exam he has hyperreflexic lower extremities, 4/5+ lower extremity muscle weakness, and stiffness in his cervical and lumbar spines. His chest expansion is normal. Which of the following best describes this patient's condition?

(A) enlarging glioma of the cerebellum
(B) large herniated lumbar disk
(C) Parkinson's disease
(D) cervical spondylosis with myelopathy
(E) Friedreich's ataxia

9. Rupture of the posterior tibial tendon can lead to

(A) inversion of the foot with heightening of the arch
(B) flattening of the arch and a valgus position of the hindfoot
(C) fixed plantar flexion of the foot
(D) fixed varus of the hindfoot
(E) fixed dorsiflexion of the foot

10. To differentiate osteoporosis from some other metabolic bone disease, which of the following laboratory tests could be obtained?

(A) glucose
(B) vitamin B_6
(C) luteinizing hormone (LH)
(D) follicle-stimulating hormone (FSH)
(E) serum protein electrophoresis

11. The biceps muscle performs which of the following?

(A) forearm flexion
(B) forearm extension
(C) forearm flexion and supination
(D) forearm flexion and pronation
(E) forearm extension and supination

12. The clinical spectrum of narcolepsy may include all of the following symptoms. Which of the symptoms refers to profound muscle weakness without loss of consciousness?

(A) disturbed nocturnal sleep
(B) cataplexy
(C) daytime somnolence
(D) hypnagogic hallucinations
(E) sleep paralysis

13. The sciatic nerve exits the sciatic notch of the pelvis beneath what muscle shown in Figure 1.1?

(A) quadratus femoris muscle
(B) gemellus muscles
(C) psoas muscle
(D) piriformis muscle
(E) posterior tibialis

14. If a pulmonary embolism (PE) is clinically suspected and the patient is symptomatic, what is the initial treatment?

(A) anticoagulation with aspirin alone
(B) anticoagulation with heparin or enoxaparin
(C) anticoagulation with Coumadin alone

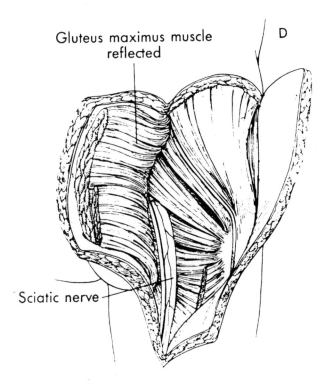

Gluteus maximus muscle reflected

D

Sciatic nerve

Figure 1.1

(D) anticoagulation must be held until an absolute diagnosis of PE is made

(E) embolectomy

15. Which of the following hormones inhibits osteoclast breakdown of bone?

(A) thyroid hormone

(B) parathyroid hormone (PTH)

(C) calcitonin

(D) corticosteroids

(E) creatine

16. Which of the following is the dominant hormonal influence on the endometrium in the proliferative phase of the menstrual cycle?

(A) estrogen

(B) progesterone

(C) testosterone

(D) cortisol

(E) testosterone

17. A 70-year-old man presents with weakness and a 30-pound weight loss over 1 year. He also has a history of vague upper abdominal

pain, back pain, and intermittent diarrhea. Physical exam reveals a cachectic-appearing man with scleral icterus. His hematocrit is 28%, with a total bilirubin of 3 mg/dL. Which of the following is the most likely diagnosis?

(A) carcinoma of the transverse colon with hepatic metastasis

(B) chronic cholecystitis with bile duct stones

(C) duodenal ulcer with pancreatic penetration

(D) carcinoma of the pancreas

(E) renal carcinoma

18. A 65-year-old patient with emphysema flies in a commercial airplane from Philadelphia to Denver. While the patient's oxygen saturation was normal in Philadelphia at rest, he becomes hypoxic during the flight. Which of the following mechanisms most likely results in the patient's hypoxemia?

(A) a decrease in the barometric air pressure

(B) ventilation–perfusion (V/Q) mismatch from underlying emphysema

(C) diffusion limitation of oxygen from interstitial scarring

(D) a decrease in the FiO_2 in the airplane cabin

(E) enhancement of shunt physiology due to altitude

19. A 34-year-old man is seen in the emergency department (ED) after having been found unresponsive by a friend. The patient is obtunded and has evidence of emesis and odor of alcohol. Track marks are noted on the forearms and antecubital fossa. The arterial blood gas shows a pH of 7.15, $PaCO_2$ of 90, and PaO_2 of 50. The patient's reduced oxygen tension is most likely due to

(A) aspiration pneumonitis following alcohol binge

(B) *Pneumocystis carinii* pneumonia (PCP) from human immunodeficiency virus (HIV)

(C) hypoventilation from narcotic overdose

(D) hypercapneic respiratory failure due to chronic obstructive pulmonary disease (COPD) exacerbation

(E) starvation ketoacidosis

20. A patient with acute respiratory distress syndrome (ARDS) on controlled mechanical ventilatory support develops progressive hypercapnea, despite a stable minute ventilation over the past several days. Which of the following interventions likely aggravated this?

(A) decreasing the respiratory rate to prevent auto–positive end-expiratory pressure (PEEP)

(B) initiation of enteral feeding for nutritional support

(C) discontinuation of steroids used initially to treat bronchospasm

(D) decreasing the tidal volume during attempts at weaning

(E) increasing sedation due to the patient's being agitated and developing ventilator dyssynchrony

21. An 85-year-old woman presents with acute onset of knee pain with swelling. Her white blood cell (WBC) count is 13,000, and her knee has a 3+ effusion and is warm to the

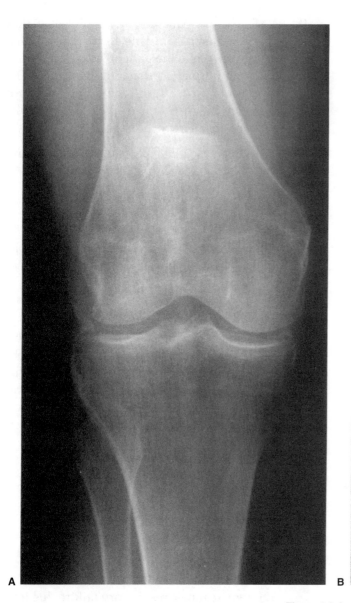

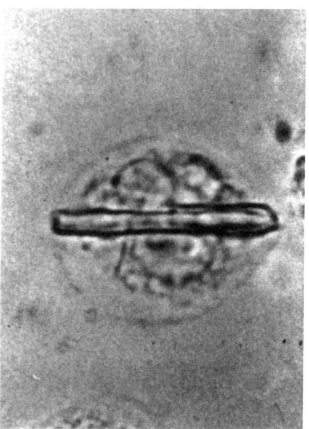

A   B

Figure 1.2 A and B
(Reproduced, with permission, from Klippel JH (ed). *Primer on the Rheumatic Diseases*, 11th ed. Atlanta, GA: Arthritis Foundation, 1997: 227 [Figure 16.2].)

touch. An x-ray of her knee and a photomicrograph of her knee aspirate are shown in Figure 1.2 A and B. Which of the following is the most likely diagnosis?

(A) septic arthritis
(B) gouty arthritis
(C) pseudogout
(D) rheumatoid arthritis
(E) Lyme arthritis

22. A 16-year-old girl is seen in an ED for increasing shortness of breath. On exam, she is tachypneic and febrile to 38.3°C (101°F), with skin pallor. Her WBC is 100,000/µL with 95% lymphoblasts. A chest x-ray is obtained showing which of the following?

(A) bilateral pleural effusions
(B) cardiomegaly
(C) a mediastinal mass
(D) right lobar pneumonia
(E) diffuse pulmonary fibrosis

23. Scurvy results from deficiency of which vitamin?

(A) vitamin A
(B) vitamin C
(C) vitamin D
(D) thiamine
(E) folate

24. A 70-year-old woman is admitted to the intensive care unit (ICU) for respiratory failure due to a severe community-acquired pneumonia. Which of the following is insignificant in affecting the shift of her oxygen–hemoglobin dissociation curve shown in Figure 1.3?

(A) acidemia
(B) hypophosphatemia
(C) fever
(D) lung consolidation
(E) pH

25. An intravenous drug user develops fever, heart murmur, and tender papules on the palms. Which of the following is the most likely diagnosis of the palmar lesions?

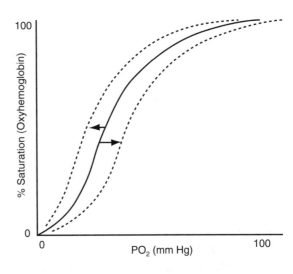

Figure 1.3

(A) Lisch nodules
(B) Osler's nodes
(C) Gottron's papules
(D) Auspitz sign
(E) Henderson-Patterson bodies

26. Figure 1.4 shows which of the following conditions?

(A) peptic ulcer disease
(B) Barrett's esophagus
(C) erosive esophagitis
(D) *Helicobacter pylori* infection
(E) normal anatomy

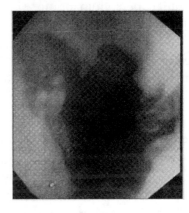

Figure 1.4
(Reproduced, with permission, from Friedman SL, McQuaid KR, Grendell JH. *Current Diagnosis & Treatment in Gastroenterology.* New York: McGraw-Hill, 2003: 278.)

27. Which of the following patients should undergo colorectal cancer screening?

    (A) a 25-year-old man with no family history of colon cancer but who notes occasional blood-streaked toilet paper
    (B) a 55-year-old man without a family history of colon cancer
    (C) an 80-year-old man with a negative colonoscopic examination 2 years ago who presents to your office requesting a repeat colonoscopy
    (D) a 35-year-old woman noted to have iron-deficiency anemia
    (E) a 17-year-old male with stomach pain

28. A 43-year-old obese diabetic woman was readmitted to the hospital for a severe wound infection following an open cholecystectomy. Despite appropriate management of the wound infection, her pain remained difficult to control, and a maintenance continuous infusion of meperidine with patient-controlled analgesia (PCA) was started. The patient and her wounds began to recover nicely when on hospital day 4 she developed seizures that were difficult to arrest. After control of her convulsions and stabilization, what is the next most appropriate step?

    (A) Obtain a magnetic resonance imaging (MRI) scan of the head with attention to the temporal lobes.
    (B) Start broad-spectrum antibiotics.
    (C) Discontinue meperidine.
    (D) Initiate phenytoin for life.
    (E) Initiate Tegretol for life.

29. Which of the following statements is true regarding the synthesis of estrogens and androgens in males?

    (A) Very little circulating testosterone is secreted from the Leydig cells of the testes.
    (B) A negligible amount of circulating dihydrotestosterone (DHT) is formed by peripheral conversion of its precursors.
    (C) The majority of circulating estradiol is not formed from peripheral conversion of its precursors.

    (D) The majority of circulating dehydroepiandrosterone sulfate (DHEAS) is secreted by the adrenals.
    (E) There is no estradiol in males.

30. A positive test for antineutrophil cytoplasmic antibody (ANCA) is most commonly found in which of the following conditions?

    (A) systemic lupus erythematosus (SLE)
    (B) Sjögren's syndrome
    (C) dermatomyositis
    (D) Wegener's granulomatosis
    (E) neurofibromatosis

31. Which of the following terms best describes a nerve injury in which structures within the perineurium and endoneurial tubes are disrupted and regeneration is disorderly?

    (A) neurotmesis
    (B) neurapraxia
    (C) axonotmesis
    (D) axesis
    (E) dermatofibrosis

32. Which of the following glands is derived from the embryonal neuroectoderm?

    (A) adrenal cortex
    (B) anterior pituitary
    (C) posterior pituitary
    (D) parathyroid glands
    (E) pancreas

33. Which disease is most likely to be associated with elevated titers of voltage-gated calcium channel antibody?

    (A) myasthenia gravis
    (B) Lambert-Eaton myasthenic syndrome
    (C) paraneoplastic polyneuropathy
    (D) myotonia congenita
    (E) Guillain-Barré syndrome

34. Which of the following immunomodulating agents used in the treatment of multiple sclerosis may exert its effect by blocking alpha-integrin?

(A) cyclosporine
(B) azathioprine
(C) mitoxantrone
(D) natalazumab
(E) glatiramer acetate

35. A 52-year-old patient has type 2 diabetes mellitus controlled with diet alone. Due to poor sugar control, a decision is made to add an oral hypoglycemic agent. Two weeks later, the patient complains of a deep aching pain over the anterior thigh and lower back. Skin is sensitive to touch over the medial thigh. Exam reveals atrophy and 3/5 weakness of the quadriceps and iliopsoas muscles, sparing the adductor magnus and all distal muscles in the leg. The knee jerk is absent on the affected side. Which nerve has been compromised?

(A) sciatic
(B) obturator
(C) femoral
(D) tibial
(E) superior gluteal

36. Which of the following is the most common anatomic lesion for the pathology associated with complex partial epilepsy?

(A) amygdala
(B) hippocampus
(C) supplementary motor cortex
(D) Purkinje cell
(E) hypothalamus

37. Which of the following would best distinguish an otherwise healthy person with severe water deprivation from a person with the syndrome of inappropriate antidiuretic hormone secretion (SIADH)?

(A) urine osmolarity
(B) plasma osmolarity
(C) circulating levels of antidiuretic hormone (ADH)
(D) corticopapillary osmotic gradient
(E) chest x-ray

38. A 40-year-old carpenter presents with a 2-cm laceration to the palm from the hooked end of a carpet knife. He is able to make a fist, and he has normal digital nerve sensation and normal capillary refill in all nail beds. When active flexion of the index and ring fingers is blocked, he is unable to flex the proximal interphalangeal joint of the long finger. Which of the following tendons has been lacerated?

(A) flexor pollicis longus
(B) flexor pollicis brevis
(C) flexor digitorum sublimis
(D) flexor digitorum profundus
(E) not a tendon injury

39. Which of the following statements about variant angina is correct?

(A) Patients with variant angina have multiple risk factors for coronary artery disease (CAD).
(B) Variant angina shows no circadian variation.
(C) Coronary arteries typically are abnormal on cardiac catheterization in patients with variant angina.
(D) Variant angina does not occur during exercise.
(E) Substance abuse such as cocaine may be an important risk factor in variant angina.

40. Which of the following drugs may produce a parkinsonian syndrome?

(A) haloperidol
(B) metoclopramide
(C) prochlorperazine
(D) amoxicillin
(E) erythromycin

41. Which of the following is an effect of PTH?

    (A) decrease in calcium reabsorption in the renal distal tubule
    (B) does not affect inhibition of phosphate reabsorption in the renal proximal tubule
    (C) stimulation of 1α-hydroxylase in the kidney
    (D) increase in serum iron
    (E) excessive axillary hair growth

42. A 40-year-old patient is being treated for acute bronchopneumonia and is doing well on antibiotics. The patient is seen by a medical student, who documents that the patient works in a ceramic factory. What further information should be ascertained?

    (A) Perform a skin test for beryllium.
    (B) Ask the patient if he ever worked in a coal mine.
    (C) Ask if the factory is old and has the potential for asbestos.
    (D) Reorder a chest x-ray to look for cavitation.
    (E) See if the patient is on steroids.

43. Lyme disease is a tick-borne illness producing an inflammatory arthritis late in the illness. It is caused by which of the following organisms?

    (A) *Borrelia burgdorferi*
    (B) *Vibrio parahaemolyticus*
    (C) *Chlamydia trachomatis*
    (D) *Pseudomonas aeruginosa*
    (E) *Enterobiasis vermiculosis*

44. Which of the following causes increased aldosterone secretion?

    (A) decreased blood volume
    (B) administration of an angiotensin-converting enzyme (ACE) inhibitor
    (C) hyperosmolarity
    (D) hypokalemia
    (E) stress

45. A 60-year-old woman presents with a 2-cm laceration to the mid-dorsum of the hand. She is able to fully extend all of her fingers; however, extension of the long finger is slightly weak. Exploration of the wound reveals the distal end of the cut extensor tendon to the long finger. How is she able to extend the long finger?

    (A) extension through the interosseus muscles
    (B) extension through the lumbrical muscles
    (C) extension through an anomalous slip from the extensor carpi radialis tendon
    (D) extension through a juncturae tendinum
    (E) "mind over matter"

46. A patient presents to his family medical doctor with a prior diagnosis of multiple endocrine neoplasia type 1 (MEN 1) for a routine medical check. Which of the following laboratory studies would be expected to be abnormal?

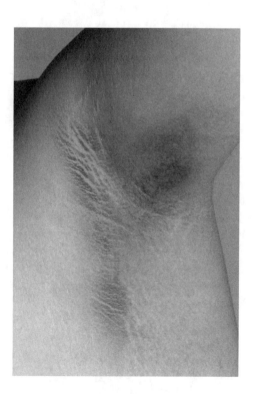

Figure 1.5
(Reproduced, with permission, from Wolff K, Johnson R, Suurmond D. *Fitzpatrick's Color Atlas & Synopsis of Clinical Dermatology.* New York: McGraw-Hill, 2005:87.)

(A) serum TSH level

(B) serum PTH level

(C) serum calcitonin level

(D) serum creatinine level

(E) serum PSA

47. In which of the following tissues are tumors likely to occur in MEN 1?

(A) ovary

(B) brain

(C) pancreas

(D) lung

(E) genital

48. A 12-year-old girl has diffuse, velvety thickening with hyperpigmentation in the axillae and sides of the neck. What underlying condition should be considered?

(A) neurofibromatosis

(B) diabetes mellitus

(C) Peutz-Jeghers syndrome

(D) SLE

(E) hypothyroidism

49. A 25-year-old obese woman presents with a rash involving her bilateral axillae (Figure 1.5). Which of the following laboratory tests would be most useful in establishing the cause?

(A) insulin

(B) hepatitis B serologies

(C) antinuclear antibody

(D) progesterone

(E) ferritin

50. A 34-year-old woman presents with a generalized rash characterized by reddish-brown, slightly raised papules extending onto the palms. What is the most likely diagnosis?

(A) psoriasis

(B) herpes simplex

(C) syphilis

(D) pityriasis rosea

(E) folliculitis

Answers and Explanations

1. **(B)** The motor weakness distribution is typical of middle cerebral artery territory. The anterior cerebral artery typically affects the contralateral leg more than the face and arm. Language deficits are usually produced by middle cerebral artery occlusions in the dominant hemisphere. Posterior artery occlusions may produce visual field defects via damage to the occipital lobe.

2. **(D)** This patient has suffered a lateral medulla stroke producing the multiple symptoms described. Basilar artery occlusions typically produce more widespread brain stem damage.

3. **(C)** Hypothyroidism leads to a very characteristic loss of the lateral third of the eyebrows, not the other conditions mentioned.

4. **(D)** The patient has Graves' disease, which is associated with pretibial myxedema. In Graves' disease, TSH is low and free T_4 is high.

5. **(B)** 1,25(OH)2D promotes the differentiation of osteoblasts. It also stimulates production of osteoclast differentiation factor (ODF), which stimulates osteoclast differentiation and activity. Estradiol suppresses various cytokines that stimulate the proliferation of osteoclast precursors. It is also associated with increased levels of osteoprotegerin, which inhibits ODF. Both calcitonin and bisphosphonates (e.g., alendronate) inhibit osteoclastic bone resorption.

6. **(B)** Squamous cell carcinoma (SCC) is a malignant neoplasm of keratinocytes. SCC of the lip usually arises from a chronically damaged epithelium secondary to sun exposure or smoking.

7. **(D)** This patient most likely has ovarian cancer. Given her age and presentation, an epithelial type of ovarian cancer is most likely and CA 125 is the tumor marker most likely to be elevated in this situation. Estradiol is elevated with the less common granulosa cell tumor. β-hCG is elevated with normal pregnancy as well as gestational trophoblastic neoplasias, including choriocarcinoma. AFP may be elevated with the less common endodermal sinus tumors, which are germ cell tumors usually diagnosed in younger women.

8. **(D)** A cerebellar tumor can produce balance problems, resulting in a wide-spaced gait. Weakness is not a key finding. A herniated lumbar disk can produce lower extremity weakness but decreased or absent deep tendon reflexes. Parkinson's disease affects the basal ganglia, producing tremor, masklike facies, cogwheel rigidity, and a shuffling gait. Weakness is not a major complaint in these patients. Friedreich's ataxia is an autosomal recessive inherited ataxia involving a mutation on chromosome 9. In general, patients with this disorder are nonambulatory by age 20. Cervical spondylosis, when severe, can result in cervical spinal stenosis severe enough to cause pyramidal tract compression and long-tract signs on examination. A decreased chest expansion implies the possibility of ankylosing spondylitis, which can result in intervertebral fusion of the entire spine and sacroiliac joints. It is seen more of-

ten in men and is associated with the presence of the histocompatability antigen HLA-B27.

9. **(B)** Chronic rupture of the posterior tibial tendon is seen commonly in elderly females. Loss of the tendon's pull on the tarsal navicular results in a gradual loss of the arch and a valgus position of the hindfoot. The patient will be unable to invert the heel on toe-standing. Valgus = out, varus = in; always look at the distal end.

10. **(E)** One could obtain a parathyroid hormone level, which, if elevated, may indicate the presence of a parathyroid adenoma. A low vitamin D level (not B_6) indicates liver or kidney disease. Multiple myeloma can be detected by a serum protein electrophoresis. Hyperthyroidism can lead to osteopenia. If these tests are normal, then a person with osteopenia probably has osteoporosis.

11. **(C)** The biceps muscle inserts on the biceps tuberosity of the proximal radius and is therefore a flexor and supinator of the forearm.

12. **(B)** Cataplexy is defined as brief, sudden episodes of muscle weakness without loss of consciousness and often triggered by an intense emotional stimulus. Hypnagogic hallucinations refer to a vivid visual dreamlike episode that commonly features the patient. During sleep paralysis, the patient is awake but is unable to move, speak, or open his or her eyes. These attacks typically occur when falling asleep or waking up.

13. **(D)** All of the muscles listed are short external rotators of the hip except the psoas muscle, which is a hip flexor and external rotator. The psoas muscle inserts on the lesser trochanter of the femur.

14. **(B)** Pulmonary embolism remains a diagnostic challenge to many physicians. First there needs to be a high clinical suspicion, and the diagnosis should be considered in certain patients presenting with symptoms such as shortness of breath, palpitations, new-onset tachycardia, and chest pain. Risk factors for venous thromboembolic disease should be considered, such as history of immobility (bed rest, recent long car or plane trips), malignancy, or family or personal history of venous thromboembolic disease. Many tests are utilized in the diagnosis of PE, inclusing pulse oximetry, ABG, EKG, CXR, D-dimer, CT scan (high-resolution CT angiography) of the chest, V/Q scan, and pulmonary angiogram.

The CT scan, done with intravenous contrast, is good for finding larger venous thromboemboli that are located in the central vessels in the lung, because the radiologist can actually see a filling defect on the CT scan. Smaller venous thromboemboli that are in the peripheral circulation can often be missed.

The D-dimer has a good negative predictive value: If it is negative, the likelihood that there is a clot is low.

When PE is suspected, treatment should be started immediately with either unfractionated or low-molecular-weight heparin. The diagnosis can be difficult, and treatment should not be withheld while testing is done.

The gold standard is a pulmonary angiogram. This procedure involves direct catheterization of the pulmonary vasculature to look for a filling defect, and is almost 100% accurate. It is, however, an invasive test and carries a risk of morbidity and mortality.

15. **(C)** Hyperparathyroidism and hyperthyroidism cause osteoporosis. Prolonged cortisone therapy and increased cortisol levels, as seen in Cushing's disease, cause osteoporosis. Calcitonin is useful in treating Paget's disease of bone and osteoporosis. It is available in an injectable form and as a nasal spray.

16. **(A)** During the proliferative phase, the predominant hormonal influence on the endometrium is estrogen. After ovulation, progesterone has the predominant influence. Testosterone and cortisol levels are fairly constant throughout the normal menstrual cycle and have no effect on the endometrium.

17. **(D)** Pancreatic carcinoma is the most likely diagnosis. The relatively short duration of symptoms and significant weight loss do not suggest a chronic condition. A penetrating ulcer would present more acutely, and weight loss would be unusual. Although metastatic colon cancer can present in a similar fashion, back pain is not usually a presenting feature.

18. **(D)** All of the choices listed are potential causes of hypoxia. In a patient with emphysema, V/Q mismatch accounts for a reduced oxygen tension, but the degree of mismatch should not have changed signficiantly as a function of altitude. The patient's becoming overtly hypoxemic during the flight, however, is due to the reduced barometric pressure. At "cabin altitude," which is pressurized to maintain equivalent atmospheric pressure at most of 8000 feet, the barometric pressure falls from 760 mmHg at sea level, to less than 600 in flight. The inspired fraction of oxygen (FiO_2) does not change significantly due to altitude. The alveolar gas equation of $PaO_2 = [FiO_2 \times (P_{atm} - P_{H20})] - (PaCO_2/R)$ reflects the contribution of each of these variables. Shunt and diffusion limitations are not primary factors for the development of hypoxia in patients with emphysema.

19. **(C)** Based on the alveolar gas equation $PaO_2 = [FiO_2 \times (P_{atm} - P_{H20})] - (PaCO_2/R)$, the patient's A-a gradient is normal. In this case, the A-a gradient is 2. Therefore, the reduced arterial oxygen tension is a consequence of the alveolar hypoventilation and the subsequent hypercarbia. The A-a gradient is normal, which suggests that there is no significant underlying parenchymal lung disease such as a pneumonia or aspiration that would explain the hypoxemia. Although COPD exacerbation can lead to hypercapneic respiratory failure, such patients have significant lung disease and would have an elevated A-a gradient. Metabolic acidosis, as with ketoacidosis, is not a direct cause of hypoxemia. The best answer given the normal

A-a gradient is that the patient is hypoventilating, most likely from narcotic abuse.

20. **(B)** Arterial $PaCO_2$ is a function of the balance between the generation and the removal of carbon dioxide. Ventilation is the primary mechanism in which the carbon dioxide is expelled, but it is important to keep in mind that carbon dioxide generation can be accelerated in certain states. These include catabolic states such as in critical illness, which can be further accelerated by steroid use. Reducing the tidal volume or the respiratory rate on the ventilator could decrease removal of carbon dioxide, but we are told that the minute ventilation (tidal volume × respiratory rate) has remained stable. The work of breathing in a patient with respiratory failure is a major source of energy expenditure and generation of carbon dioxide; therefore, the addition of sedation to decrease the dyssynchrony with the ventilator and the work of breathing may aid in limiting hypercarbia. Intuitively, oversedation may decrease ventilation, leading to hypercarbia, but again, the patient is mechanically ventilated and the minute ventilation has been stable. The best answer is that initiation of nutritional support, which is critical to patients with prolonged critical illness, has contributed to increased metabolism and generation of carbon dioxide.

21. **(C)** Pseudogout can present like septic arthritis with fever and an increased WBC count and erythrocyte sedimentation rate. An acute gouty attack can present in a similar manner. Calcium pyrophosphate dihydrate crystals are deposited in articular cartilage and appear on x-ray as radiodensities known as chondrocalcinosis. Deposition of crystals can be seen in the menisci and articular cartilage in the x-ray in Figure 1.3. Calcium pyrophosphate crystals are rod shaped. Urate crystals in gout are needle shaped. Nonsteroidal anti-inflammatory agents are the treatment of choice for pseudogout.

22. **(C)** The patient most likely has acute lymphoblastic leukemia or lymphoma with a

thymic mass. This patient could have a concurrent infection that is not the cause of her respiratory distress. Pleural effusions can occur but not usually initially. Neither cardiomegaly nor pulmonary fibrosis have any relevance in this case.

23. **(B)** Vitamin C is essential for normal collagen metabolism. Deficiency of vitamin C (scurvy) results in impairment of wound healing and perifollicular hemorrhage.

24. **(D)** Although lung consolidation has a significant effect on ventilation and perfusion, leading to disturbances in gas exchange, it does not directly contribute to shifts in the oxygen–hemoglobin dissociation curve. The three most important factors that affect the oxygen–hemoglobin dissociation curve are pH, temperature, and 2,3-DPG (2-3-diphosphoglycerate). Pyrexia, acidemia, and increases in 2,3-DPG all act to shift the curve to the right. The net effect of a rightward shift is to enhance dissociation of oxygen from hemoglobin at a given oxygen tension (PaO_2).

25. **(B)** Osler's nodes are tender palmar papules arising in the setting of bacterial endocarditis. They may be caused by minute infective emboli or immunologic phenomena, resulting in small-vessel vasculitis.

26. **B)** The photograph depicted is that of an endoscopic image taken of the lower esophagus. One can identify the normal-appearing esophageal mucosa and the overlying salmon tongues of metaplastic tissue characteristic of Barrett's esophagus. Since no ulceration is identified, peptic ulcer disease is not possible. There is no evidence of either erosive esophagitis or *H. pylori* infection.

27. **(B)** It is recommended that any adult over the age of 50 undergo screening for colorectal cancer. If a colonoscopy is performed and is normal, then a repeat colonoscopy can be performed in 5 to 10 years for additional screening. The most likely cause of blood-streaked toilet paper in a young patient is hemorrhoids, and an anoscopic examination would be sufficient to document this. Iron deficiency in a premenopausal woman is not likely to be caused by a colonic source.

28. **(C)** Meperidine has traditionally been used in surgical cases involving the biliary tree as it is suspected to cause less of a spasm on the sphincter of Oddi than other traditional opiates. Smooth-muscle contractions occur to a lesser extent, and urinary retention is less compared to morphine. Pupil dilation rather than constriction occurs with meperidine, unlike other opiates (due to an atropine-like activity). However, meperidine is metabolized by the liver to normeperidine and is excreted in the urine. With excessive use, the metabolites are neurotoxic and can lead to tremors, myoclonus, and even seizures, possibly potentiated by any existing renal failure. Therefore, an appropriate next step in this patient who had been recovering nicely is to discontinue meperidine.

29. **(D)** DHEAS is secreted primarily by the adrenal gland. The majority of circulating testosterone is secreted by the testicular Leydig cells. DHT and estradiol are formed primarily by peripheral conversion of testosterone and other precursors.

30. **(D)** A positive ANCA is seen in Wegener's granulomatosis. Postitivity correlates well with disease activity. ANCA is not uniquely seen in this disease.

31. **(A)** Neurapraxia involves loss of conduction across a damaged segment. The axons are not disrupted, and wallerian degeneration does not occur. Recovery is spontaneous and complete. Axonotmesis involves axonal disruption and wallerian degeneration of the axon distal to the injury site. The Schwann cell sheath is not disrupted and serves as a guide for the regenerating axon. In neurotmesis, regeneration is disorderly, and reinnervation occurs at a speed of 1 mm per day. The more distal the injury, the better the result. Any injury greater than this requires surgical repair.

32. **(C)** The posterior pituitary gland is derived from the neuroectoderm, while the anterior pituitary arises from surface ectoderm. The adrenal cortex originates from mesoderm. Both the parathyroids and the pancreas originate from endoderm.

33. **(B)** In the Lambert-Eaton syndrome an autoantibody attacks the presynaptic membrane of the neuromuscular junction. It is commonly associated with an underlying neoplasm (e.g., small cell lung cancer) and presents with proximal muscle weakness, autonomic dysfunction, and bulbar weakness without ptosis or extraocular motility disorder. Forty percent of patients may present without an underlying neoplasm.

34. **(D)** Natalazumab is the first selective adhesion molecule inhibitor to become available. It acts by preventing the entry of inflammatory cells into the central nervous system at the vascular level. Initial studies have demonstrated a decrease in relapse rate of greater than 60%.

35. **(C)** Diabetic amyotrophy commonly appears at the time of acute hyperglycemia or after treatment of hyperglycemia. It frequently will later affect the contralateral side. There is always associated pain and often allodynia in the distribution of the femoral nerve. It is a self-limited condition but the pain can be quite debilitating and often requires acute immunosuppression for pain relief. The quadriceps and iliopsoas muscles are supplied by the femoral nerve. The sparing of the adductor magnus makes an obturator neuropathy unlikely, and the sparing of the tibialis anterior is against an L4 root localization.

36. **(B)** Mesial temporal sclerosis is commonly seen pathologically in the hypothalamus of patients with complex partial epilepsy. In later-onset seizure disorders, neoplasm and cerebral infarction are the most common etiologies.

37. **(B)** Both individuals will have hyperosmotic urine, a normal corticopapillary gradient, and high circulating levels of ADH. The person with water deprivation will have a high plasma osmolarity, and the person with SIADH will have a low plasma osmolarity.

38. **(C)** The flexor digitorum sublimis tendons are superficial to the profundus tendons in the palm and the palmar aspect of the proximal phalanges of the index, long, ring, and little fingers. Over the proximal phalanx, the sublimis tendon splits to allow passage of the profundus tendon through it. The sublimis tendon inserts on the middle phalanx as two slips. The profundus tendon inserts on the palmar aspect of the distal phalanx.

39. **(E)** In general, patients with variant angina are younger and do not have multiple risk factors for CAD, although cigarette smoking may play a role. Patients with variant angina may have other vasospastic disorders like Raynaud's. Episodes of spasm tend to occur more frequently from midnight to early morning. Substance abuse may play an important role, and, with cocaine abuse, coronary spasm may lead to myocardial infarction despite normal coronary arteries as seen at angiogram. Although there is a circadian pattern to episodes of chest pain, exercise can precipitate attacks of vasospastic or variant angina.

40. **(B)** Metoclopramide, a medication used commonly for gastric motility abnormalities, will commonly produce a parkinsonian syndrome. The phenothiazines, even when not used for their antipsychotic properties (e.g., for nausea or cough) will still readily produce extrapyramidal signs.

41. **(C)** PTH stimulates 1α-hydroxylase in the kidney. This enzyme converts 25-hydroxyvitamin D into its active metabolite, 1,25-dihydroxyvitamin D. PTH maintains serum calcium levels by increasing osteoclastic activity and increasing calcium reabsorption in the distal renal tubule. It regulates serum phosphate levels by inhibiting phosphate reabsorption in the renal proximal tubule.

42. **(A)** Exposure to beryllium dust can cause acute bronchopneumonia. Asbestosis does not present as bronchopneumonia but as interstitial disease. Steroids can cause an immunosuppressive state. Coal miners can develop bronchopneumonia but in general tend to develop severe emphysema or lung cancer.

43. **(A)** Lyme disease is characterized by three stages. Stage 1 is a localized infection at the site of the tick bite. Stage 2 occurs within 3 to 32 days with characteristic skin lesions, erythema migrans, and migratory muscle pain. Stage 3 occurs at 6 months postinfection with intermittent mono- or oligoarthritis of large joints. Amoxicillin is effective in early stages of the disease.

44. **(A)** Decreased blood volume stimulates secretion of renin and initiates the renin–angiotensin–aldosterone axis for stimulation of aldosterone secretion. ACE inhibitors block this axis by decreasing production of antithrombin II. Hyperosmolarity stimulates ADH secretion. Hyperkalemia has a direct effect on the adrenal cortex to stimulate aldosterone secretion.

45. **(D)** Juncturae connect the tendons of the extensor digitorum communis at the level of the metacarpal heads. Multiple variations have been observed; however, the extensor digitorum communis (EDC) tendon to the long finger is almost always included.

46. **(B)** In patients with MEN 1, the characteristic test that is elevated is the serum PTH. In patients with this syndrome, the development of either pituitary, parathyroid, or pancreatic endocrine tumors is possible. The serum TSH level is normal in these patients. The serum calcitonin level may be elevated in patients with MEN 2 and predicts the development of a medullary thyroid tumor. The serum creatinine is normal in patients with MEN 1.

47. **(C)** As described above, patients with MEN 1 may develop pancreatic endocrine tumors. Ovarian, brain, genital, and lung tumors are not characteristically seen with this syndrome.

48. **(B)** Acanthosis nigricans is characterized by symmetric hyperpigmentation and papillary hypertrophy of the neck, axillae, groin, and other flexor surfaces. It is frequently associated with an underlying endocrinopathy, including diabetes mellitus.

49. **(A)** Figure 1.5 depicts acanthosis nigricans, characterized by hyperpigmentation and papillary hypertrophy. Rash is generally symmetrically distributed, and common locations are the axillae, neck, medial thighs, and groin. The most common variety of acanthosis nigricans occurs in the setting of insulin-resistant states and obesity.

50. **(C)** Secondary syphilis may present with bilateral, symmetric, nonpruritic macules followed by red papular lesions involving the face, scalp, palms, and soles.

Practice Test 2
Questions

DIRECTIONS (Questions 1 through 50): Each of the numbered items or incomplete statements in this section is followed by answers or by completions of the statement. Select the ONE answer or completion that is BEST in each case.

1. What peripheral blood abnormality is commonly found in patients with atopic dermatitis?

   (A) leukocytosis
   (B) anemia
   (C) eosinophilia
   (D) thrombocytopenia
   (E) increased lactic dehydrogenase (LDH)

2. Sarcoidosis is characterized histologically by which of the following features?

   (A) granulomas
   (B) increased number of melanocytes
   (C) atypical mitotic figures
   (D) necrosis
   (E) vasculitis

3. Patients with diffuse esophageal spasm (DES) are likely to have which of the following symptoms?

   (A) nausea and vomiting
   (B) atypical chest pain
   (C) diarrhea
   (D) gastroesophageal reflux disease (GERD)
   (E) hiccups

4. A necrotic ulceration of the lower extremity in a patient with ulcerative colitis most likely represents

   (A) a Shagreen patch
   (B) erythema nodosum
   (C) a tuberous xanthoma
   (D) pyoderma gangrenosum
   (E) necrobiosis lipoidica diabeticorum

5. A patient presents to the emergency department (ED) shortly after the accidental ingestion of lye. There is no evidence of esophageal perforation and the patient is managed conservatively. Which of the following is a possible long-term sequela?

   (A) GERD
   (B) gastric bezoar
   (C) esophageal stricture
   (D) gastric ulcers
   (E) pale-colored stools

6. A 29-year-old woman with asthma is being treated with supraphysiologic doses of glucocorticoids. Which of the following would she be expected to exhibit?

   (A) decreased gluconeogenesis
   (B) decreased lipolysis in adipose tissue
   (C) decreased amino acid release from muscle
   (D) elevated corticotropin (ACTH)
   (E) increased glycogen synthesis

7. A 50-year-old man presents with a several-month history of vague midepigastric abdominal pain and increasing fatigue. He also noted worsening shortness of breath with exertion. A complete blood count (CBC) was obtained with a hemoglobin of 10.5. His peripheral smear is shown in Figure 2.1. This is most consistent with

(A) spherocytosis
(B) thalassemia
(C) macrocytosis due to vitamin B_{12} deficiency
(D) iron deficiency
(E) anemia of chronic disease

8. Which of the following is most consistent with cardiogenic shock?

(A) blood pressure 85/50 mmHg, heart rate 105 beats per minute, respiratory rate 18 per minute, pulmonary capillary wedge pressure 24 mmHg
(B) blood pressure 85/50 mmHg, heart rate 105 beats per minute, respiratory rate 18 per minute, pulmonary capillary wedge pressure 6 mmHg
(C) blood pressure 85/50 mmHg, heart rate 80 beats per minute, respiratory rate 12 per minute, pulmonary capillary wedge pressure 18 mmHg
(D) blood pressure 85/50 mmHg, heart rate 80 beats per minute, respiratory rate 12 per minute, pulmonary capillary wedge pressure 12 mmHg

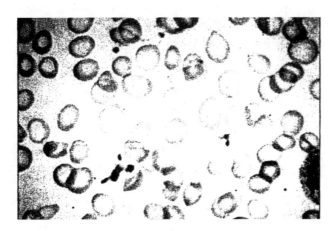

Figure 2.1

(E) blood pressure 122/84 mmHg, heart rate 80 beats per minute, respiratory rate 13 per minute, pulmonary capillary wedge normal

9. The development of antibiotic-resistant bacterial strains is facilitated by

(A) careful selection and use of antibiotics
(B) inadequate phagocytes
(C) tissue permeability
(D) plasmid transfer from resistant bacteria to antibiotic-sensitive bacteria
(E) narrow-spectrum antibiotics use

10. In which of the following early post–myocardial infarction (MI) settings would you avoid giving atropine?

(A) treatment of sinus bradycardia with low cardiac output and peripheral hypoperfusion or frequent premature ventricular contractions
(B) acute inferior infarction with type I second- or third-degree atrioventricular (AV) block associated with symptoms of hypotension, ischemic discomfort, or ventricular arrhythmias
(C) bradycardia and hypotension after administration of nitroglycerin
(D) type II AV block and third-degree AV block with new wide QRS complex due to acute MI
(E) bradycardia and PVCs

11. Regarding the use of atropine, which of the following statements is correct?

(A) The recommended dosage of atropine for bradycardia is 0.5 to 1.0 mg intravenously (IV), repeated if needed every 3 to 5 minutes to a total dose of no more than 2.5 mg (0.03 to 0.04 mg/kg).
(B) For ventricular asystole the recommended dose is 2 mg IV, to be repeated every 3 to 5 minutes (while cardiopulmonary resuscitation [CPR] continues) if asystole persists.
(C) For asystole, the total cumulative dose should not exceed 5 mg over 2.5 hours.

(D) The peak action of atropine given intravenously is observed within 20 minutes.

(E) Overdose with atropine is impossible.

12. Which of the following would be a poor choice in the treatment of neuropathic pain?

(A) amitriptyline

(B) carbamazepine

(C) gabapentin

(D) oxycodone

(E) topiramate

13. A 56-year-old man undergoes thyroidectomy for a 3-cm thyroid nodule. A fine-needle aspiration biopsy revealed a suspicious cytology, which prompted the surgery. On final pathology, which of the following features will help distinguish follicular adenoma from carcinoma?

(A) nuclear inclusions

(B) Hurthle cells

(C) spindle cells

(D) capsular invasion

(E) lymphocytes

14. The "triptan" group of antimigraine medications are primarily active at which central nervous system (CNS) receptor?

(A) beta-adrenergic

(B) alpha-adrenergic

(C) NMDA (*N*-methyl-D-aspartate)

(D) serotonergic

(E) cholinergic

15. Which of the following conditions is insignificant in the potential for increasing risk of developing cervical cancer?

(A) multiple sexual partners

(B) history of human papillomavirus (HPV) infection

(C) cigarette smoking

(D) alcohol abuse

(E) early age at first intercourse

16. Which of the following statements is true regarding the anatomy of the adrenal gland?

(A) The inferior phrenic artery supplies both adrenal glands.

(B) The adrenal cortex is poorly vascularized.

(C) The right adrenal vein drains into the right renal vein.

(D) The adrenal medulla originates from mesoderm.

(E) The zona glomerulosa is the innermost layer of the adrenal cortex.

17. What is the most common type of testicular germ cell tumor?

(A) teratoma

(B) embryonal cell tumor

(C) seminoma

(D) choriocarcinoma

(E) yolk sac tumor

18. A patient presents with an acute MI. For which of the following conditions would you withhold placement of transcutaneous pacer patches?

(A) sinus bradycardia with hypotension

(B) Mobitz type II second-degree AV block

(C) third-degree heart block

(D) bilateral bundle branch block (BBB)

(E) uncomplicated acute MI without evidence of conduction system disease

19. A 21-year-old man presents with a palpable abdominal mass, jaundice, and anemia. A chest x-ray revealed a "shell-like" calcification in the abdomen. Which of the following is the most likely diagnosis?

(A) mesoblastic nephroma

(B) neuroblastoma

(C) Wilms' tumor

(D) adrenal hemorrhage

(E) renal cell carcinoma

20. Regarding class IA antiarrhythmic drugs, which of the following statements is true?

(A) They prolong action potential duration.

(B) They reduce the maximum velocity of the action potential upstroke.

(C) They prolong conduction through the AV node.

(D) They block slow inward calcium channel current.

(E) No contraindications exist.

21. A male infant is born with a deficiency in the enzyme 11α-hydroxylase. Which of the following may result from this condition?

(A) an elevated plasma renin level

(B) hypertension

(C) small adrenal glands

(D) hyperkalemia

(E) decreased ACTH secretion

22. Which of the following antibodies is most specific for systemic lupus erythematosus (SLE)?

(A) double-stranded DNA

(B) antihistone

(C) Ro(SSA)/La(SSB)

(D) single-stranded DNA (deoxyribonucleic acid)

(E) anticentromere

23. A new blood test has been developed to diagnose prostate cancer. It has a sensitivity and specificity of 90% and 75%, respectively. What is the positive predictive value of the test if the prevalence of cancer in the group being tested is 5000 per 100,000?

(A) 10%

(B) 16%

(C) 90%

(D) 84%

(E) 99%

24. A 43-year-old man is found down and brought in by the police. He is disheveled, and a smell of alcohol is evident. His chemistries reveal the following: Na 130, K

3.4, Cl 80, HCO_3 20. An osmlolar gap is calculated and is found to be elevated. A urinalysis is significant for the presence of oxalate crystals. What is the likely diagnosis for this patient?

(A) alcohol intoxication

(B) ethylene glycol ingestion

(C) diabetic ketoacidosis

(D) salicylate ingestion

(E) methanol ingestion

25. A new sedative–hypnotic drug is released for use as a continuous infusion for patients on a mechanical ventilator. Its half-life is approximately 30 minutes. If no loading dose is given, how long will a continuous IV infusion of this medication take to reach 90% of its final steady-state level?

(A) 15 minutes

(B) 30 minutes

(C) 60 minutes

(D) 100 minutes

(E) 150 minutes

26. A 30-year-old woman presents with shaking, sweating, and dizziness. Which of the following conditions is associated with hypoglycemia and a low C peptide level?

(A) insulinoma

(B) glucagonoma

(C) somatostatinoma

(D) Cushing syndrome

(E) exogenous insulin intake

27. Which of the following hormones contributes most to insulin resistance in pregnancy?

(A) estrogen

(B) progesterone

(C) human chorionic gonadotropin (hCG)

(D) human placental lactogen

(E) prolactin

28. Cystic fibrosis is an autosomal recessive disease. It is now possible to screen for cystic fibrosis carrier status. The frequency of heterozygote carriers in the U.S. population of

European Caucasian descent is 1 in 30. What is the chance that a couple of European Caucasian descent will both be carriers?

(A) 1 in 30
(B) 1 in 60
(C) 1 in 90
(D) 1 in 300
(E) 1 in 900

29. Which of the following is the most common malignancy associated with the malignant variant of acanthosis nigricans?

(A) colon
(B) lung
(C) prostate
(D) breast
(E) stomach

30. A 60-year-old man develops acute arthritis of his left knee. An x-ray reveals chondrocalcinosis. An effusion is evident on clinical exam and is aspirated. Cell counts reveal leukocytes greater than 20,000/cc, with 90% being neutrophils. Compensated polarized microscopy reveals the presence of weakly positive birefringent crystals. Which of the following is the most likely diagnosis?

(A) pseudogout
(B) gout
(C) rheumatoid arthritis
(D) septic arthritis
(E) traumatic effusion

31. Which of the following statements concerning radiation is true?

(A) Cartilage and muscle tissue are radiosensitive.
(B) The marrow and lymphoid system are the least radiosensitive tissues of the body.
(C) A testicular germ cell tumor may be cured with radiation.
(D) Postradiation sarcomas may develop after 3 months.
(E) One thousand rads of total body radiation is safe and common at "tanning salons."

32. A 27-year-old woman presents with palpitations, tremors, anxiety, and neck pain. Her thyroid-stimulating hormone (TSH) is low and free thyroxine (T_4) is high, consistent with primary hyperthyroidism. A 24-hour radioiodine uptake is low. How would you treat this patient?

(A) methimazole
(B) radioiodine
(C) surgery
(D) propranolol
(E) oral contraceptives

33. Compression of which of the following nerves in Guyon's canal at the wrist can result in an "intrinsic minus" hand?

(A) ulnar nerve
(B) median nerve
(C) radial nerve
(D) musculocutaneous nerve
(E) peroneal nerve

34. Which immunoglobulin (Ig) can be passively transferred in utero, conferring immunity against infection such as varicella?

(A) IgA
(B) IgG
(C) IgD
(D) IgE
(E) IgM

35. A young boy presents with a rash around the eyes and on the extremities that is suspicious for dermatomyositis. Which of the following laboratory studies would most likely confirm the diagnosis?

(A) serum creatine kinase
(B) thyroid function assay
(C) lupus band
(D) 24-hour urine uroporphyrin excretion
(E) antineutrophil cytoplasmic antibody

36. A 7-year-old boy has the following clinical findings on physical examination: anividia, hemihypertrophy, and hematomas. Which of the following pediatric neoplasms is most commonly associated with the findings?

    (A) embryonal carcinoma
    (B) Wilms' tumor
    (C) neuroblastoma
    (D) adrenal carcinoma
    (E) pheochromocytoma

37. The first dorsal compartment of the wrist contains which of the following tendons?

    (A) extensor carpi radialis longus
    (B) extensor digitorum communis
    (C) extensor carpi ulnaris
    (D) abductor pollicis longus
    (E) extensor pollicis longus

38. Cellular changes suggestive of HPV infection include which of the following?

    (A) koilocytosis
    (B) multinucleated giant cell
    (C) granuloma development
    (D) plasma cell infiltration
    (E) plasma cell reduction

39. A 24-month-old boy presents with a left side abdominal mass crossing the midline, and proptosis and periorbital edema. Which of the following is the most likely diagnosis?

    (A) pheochromocytoma
    (B) rhabdosarcoma
    (C) Wilms' tumor with bone metastases
    (D) mesoblastic nephroma
    (E) neuroblastoma with bone metastases

40. A 46-year-old woman asks you to screen her for diabetes mellitus because of a strong family history. Her fasting plasma glucose is 106 mg/dL and 108 mg/dL on two separate days. She most likely has

    (A) diabetes
    (B) impaired glucose tolerance
    (C) impaired fasting glucose

    (D) normal glucose
    (E) hypoglycemia

41. Which of the following is a sexually active woman's greatest risk for developing invasive cervical cancer?

    (A) having multiple sexual partners
    (B) having a history of infection with the herpesvirus
    (C) never having Pap smear screening
    (D) having a history of cervical intraepithelial neoplasia (CIN)-2 treated with loop excision of the transformation zone with clear margins on pathology
    (E) smoking

42. The synthesis of the hormone pictured in Figure 2.2 is catalyzed by adrenocortical enzymes, including P450c17 (17α-hydroxylase) and P450c11β (11β-hydroxylase). Which adrenal zones produce this hormone?

    (A) zona fasciculata and zona reticularis
    (B) zona glomerulosa
    (C) zona remoris
    (D) zona pellucida
    (E) cortisol zone

43. Tamoxifen use as an adjunctive chemotherapeutic agent in the treatment of breast cancers is associated with an increased risk of

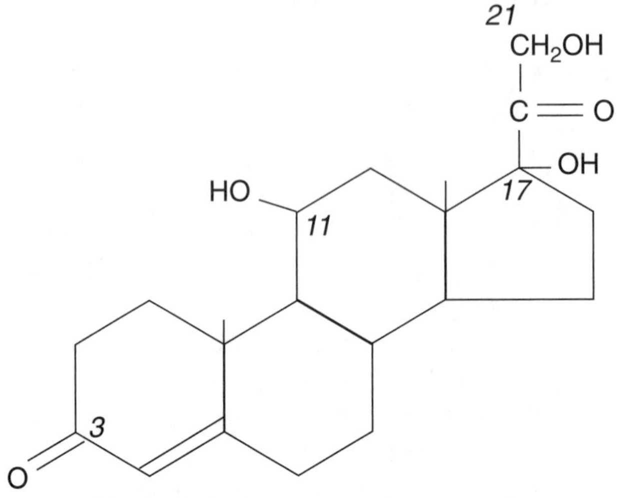

Figure 2.2

(A) cervical cancer

(B) osteoporosis

(C) heart disease

(D) endometrial cancer

(E) diabetes

44. A screening test is developed to identify hearing difficulties in infants. It is first tried in two separate hospitals. However, among those who tested positive with this new test, the rate of false-positive tests at hospital A are significantly lower than the rate at hospital B. What is the likely explanation for this discrepancy?

(A) The specificity of the test is lower in hospital B.

(B) The sensitivity of the test is lower in hospital A.

(C) The prevalence of disease is higher in hospital A.

(D) cannot be determined

(E) error in measurement

45. When leuprolide, a gonadotropin-releasing hormone (GnRH) agonist, is administered in appropriate doses, which of the following occurs?

(A) ovulation induction

(B) amenorrhea

(C) reliable contraception

(D) regulation of menstruation in patients with oligo-ovulation

(E) pregnancy

46. A 35-year-old asymptomatic female who is 6 months pregnant is referred to you for an elevated total T_4 level. Her TSH and free thyroxine (free T_4) levels are normal. Her physical exam is unremarkable. Which of the following mechanisms most likely explains these findings?

(A) TSH-secreting pituitary tumor

(B) elevated levels of thyroid-binding globulin (TBG)

(C) Graves' disease

(D) iodine deficiency

(E) thyroid carcinoma

47. Which factor is the most significant influence on increasing an individual's resting ventilatory response?

(A) hypercapnea ($PaCO_2$ of 50 mmHg)

(B) hyperoxygenation (PaO_2 of 200 mmHg)

(C) mild hypoxemia (PaO_2 of 63 mmHg)

(D) hypocapnea ($PaCO_2$ of 30 mmHg)

(E) very mild hypoxemia

48. A 54-year-old patient with cryptogenic cirrhosis is admitted for hypoxemia with a saturation of 83% on room air. The patient has no history of lung disease, and the chest radiograph is unremarkable. His saturation improves little with oxygen supplementation, but does improve in the supine position. Where in Figure 2.3 is the patient's ventilation–perfusion (V/Q) status?

(A) A

(B) B

(C) C

(D) D

(E) E

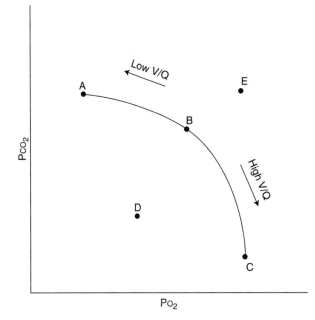

Figure 2.3

49. A 300-pound woman is brought to your office by her husband for excessive daytime hypersomnolence, significant snoring, and occasional apneic episodes noted during sleep. The respiratory pattern is measured at the thoracic and abdominal levels by elastic bands during a sleep study. Which of the patterns in Figure 2.4 would suggest obstructive sleep apnea?

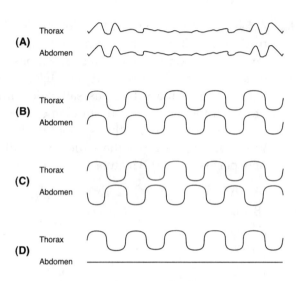

Figure 2.4 A, B, C, and D

50. Increased sebaceous gland activity is associated with

   (A) acne
   (B) atopic dermatitis
   (C) hyperhidrosis
   (D) tinea
   (E) psoriasis

Answers and Explanations

1. **(C)** Interleukin-5 (IL-5) is responsible for eosinophil differentiation. In atopic dermatitis the TH_2 phenotype predominates, with resultant IL-4, IL-5, and IL-10 production.

2. **(A)** Histologic examination of sarcoidosis reveals sparse lymphocytic infiltrate concentrated peripherally around noncaseating epithelioid granulomas.

3. **(B)** It has been a common clinical response to attribute unexplained chest pain to "esophageal spasm." In patients with a manometric pattern of DES, those presenting with chest pain have higher amplitudes than those presenting with dysphagia. Approximately one third of patients with DES show associated abnormalities of lower esophageal sphincter function, either high resting pressure or incomplete relaxation. Nausea, vomiting, and diarrhea are not considered part of the constellation of symptoms associated with DES. Similarly, patients with this motility disorder do not appear to be more likely to develop GERD.

4. **(D)** Pyoderma gangrenosum is a gangrenous ulcerative lesion that most commonly occurs on the legs in persons with ulcerative colitis.

5. **(C)** Ingestion of caustic substances such as lye is usually accidental. It occurs more commonly in children under the age of 5 and is generally due to psychiatric causes in adults and adolescents. The most common cause is ingestion of a strong alkali (sodium or potassium hydroxide) such as those contained in household cleaning products (e.g., drain cleaners) or batteries. Ingestion of alkaline substances results in a rapid, penetrating form of injury leading to liquefactive necrosis. The injury extends rapidly (within seconds) through the mucosa and wall of the esophagus and can result in penetration and perforation of the esophagus. Long-term sequelae include the development of esophageal strictures. The likelihood that a patient will develop esophageal strictures depends in part on the depth of damage and degree of collagen deposition.

6. **(E)** Glucocorticoids stimulate glycogen synthase and inhibit the breakdown of glycogen. They increase hepatic gluconeogenesis, increase lipolysis in adipose tissue, decrease protein synthesis, and increase amino acid release in muscle. Supraphysiologic doses of glucocorticoids inhibit the hypothalamic–pituitary axis, leading to suppression of ACTH levels.

7. **(D)** This smear is typical of a microcytic, hypochromic anemia occurring in those with iron deficiency. This invariably is due to chronic blood loss in this patient. The patient will obviously require a more extensive gastrointestinal evaluation since men and postmenopausal women should not present with iron-deficiency anemia. Hypochromic anemias can indeed be seen in thalassemia but usually not in the setting of midepigastric pain. Ten percent of patients with anemia of chronic disease have a microcytic anemia, but usually (90%) they present with a normochromic, normocytic picture.

8. **(A)** Cardiogenic shock arises as a result of heart pump failure and may result from myocardial infarction or other cardiac catastrophes such as severe valve dysfunction, cardiac tamponade, or massive pulmonary embolism. The patient described in choice B likely is demonstrating hypovolemic shock as evidenced by the low pulmonary capillary wedge pressure. The patient described in choice C likely has chronic heart failure, as evidenced by the pulmonary capillary wedge pressure of 18, but does not show signs of compromise as evidenced by the normal pulse and the lack of tachypnea. The patient described in choice D likely has a normal blood volume and cardiac status despite the relatively low blood pressure. The heart rate, respiratory rate, and wedge pressure are normal. The patient in choice E is normal.

9. **(D)** Plasmids contain small, independently reproducing strands of DNA (deoxyribonucleic acid) encoding proteins that alter surface receptors, change cell wall permeability, or enhance bacterial metabolism of an antibiotic itself. Proper antibiotic selection should be based on cultures and antibiotic sensitivity tests. Narrow-spectrum antibiotics decrease the risk of developing resistance.

10. **(D)** Atropine has parasympatholytic (anticholinergic) activity and reduces vagal tone. This results in an enhanced rate of discharge of the sinus node and AV conduction. Atropine is rarely used to treat type II second-degree AV block. If heart block is present distal to the AV node by increasing the sinus rate, atropine may enhance the block.

11. **(A)** The dose for ventricular asystole is 1 mg IV, to be repeated every 3 to 5 minutes (while CPR continues) if asystole persists. The total cumulative dose should not exceed 2.5 mg over 2.5 hours. Atropine has a rapid onset of action, and the peak action of atropine given intravenously is observed within 3 minutes.

12. **(D)** The opiate narcotic class of medications has not shown proven benefit in the treatment of neuropathic pain. Gabapentin, topiramate, and most of the new "anticonvulsant" medications have shown significant benefit in the the treatment of the burning, electric shock, and hyperesthetic pain associated with neuropathic pain.

13. **(D)** Capsular or vascular invasion will help distinguish follicular adenoma from carcinoma, not the other features mentioned in the question.

14. **(D)** In addition to decreasing the pain, they may also help to alleviate the nausea and vomiting associated with migraine.

15. **(D)** While all of the other factors have been associated with the development of cervical dysplasia and subsequent cancer development, alcohol abuse has not been shown to be a risk factor.

16. **(A)** The adrenal cortices are well vascularized, and both receive their main arterial supply from the inferior phrenic artery, the renal arteries, and the aorta. A single central vein drains each gland. The right adrenal vein drains into the vena cava, whereas the left adrenal vein drains into the left renal vein. The adrenal cortex originates from mesoderm, but the adrenal medulla is derived from neuroectoderm. The cortex is comprised of three layers: the outer zona glomerulosa, the zona fasciculata, and the inner zona reticularis.

17. **(C)** Seminomas are the most common of the testicular tumors, accounting for more than 70% of germ cell neoplasms of the testis. Teratomas are the second most common. Yolk sac tumors, choriocarcinomas, and embryonal cell tumors occur much less frequently.

18. **(E)** All of the other conditions may lead to worsened AV conduction and more severe bradycardia.

19. **(D)** Adrenal hemorrhages are found in 1% to 2% of neonates undergoing autopsy. The initial presentation is particularly difficult to

distinguish from hemorrhage within a neuroblastoma. The clinical presentation includes signs of blood loss, sepsis, shock, and the presence of an abdominal mass. "Shell"-like calcifications occur late or following recovery.

20. **(A)** Reduction of the maximum velocity of the action potential upstroke is characteristic of type Ib antiarrhythmics. Prolonged conduction through the AV node is a property associated with class II or beta blockers. Slow inward calcium channel current blockade is associated with class IV or calcium channel blockers.

21. **(B)** A deficiency in 11α-hydroxylase leads to cortisol deficiency and an excess of 11-deoxycorticosterone, 11-deoxycortisol, and adrenal androgens. The cortisol deficiency will stimulate increased secretion of ACTH and therefore adrenal gland hypertrophy. The 11- deoxycorticosterone has mineralocorticoid effects, and excess levels may lead to hypertension, hypokalemia, and suppression of renin. The elevated adrenal androgen levels may lead to virilization in females but would not have a significant effect on males.

22. **(A)** Double-stranded DNA antibodies are highly specific for SLE.

23. **(B)** A 2 × 2 table should be constructed as follows: The prevalence is the rate of disease in the given population and is listed in the final row. Knowing that the sensitivity is a/(a + c) and that specificity is d/(b + d), the table can be subsequently filled out. The *positive predictive value* can then be calculated as a/(a + b) and reflects the percentage that a positive test accurately identifies the presence of the true disease (prostate cancer). Note the dependence of the positive predictive value on both the prevalence of disease and the specificity of the test.

	Prostate Cancer	No Prostate Cancer	
Test Positive	4500 (a)	23,750 (b)	28,250
Test Negative	500 (c)	71,250 (d)	71,750
	5000	95,000	100,000

24. **(B)** In unresponsive patients, the calculation of the *anion gap* and osmolar gap are important in considering possible ingestions. In this patient, there is a significant "gapped" metabolic acidosis as marked by an anion gap of 30 ($AG = Na - Cl - HCO_3$). This suggests the presence of excessive anions. These anions, or rather the differential for an anion-gapped metabolic acidosis, includes diabetic ketoacidosis, methanol ingestion, uremia, lactic acidosis, ethylene glycol ingestion, and salicylate overdose. However, the presence of an osmolar gap—the difference between the measured and calculated serum osmolality—suggests an anion gap typically resulting from ingestion of either methanol or ethylene glycol, although several others can cause an increase in the gap (> 10). Regardless, however, the presence of oxaluria is specific for ethylene glycol ingestion in this case, as ethylene glycol is metabolized to oxalic acid, just as methanol would be metabolized to formic acid. The oxaluria can further lead to oxalate stone precipitation and cause acute renal failure.

25. **(D)** Understanding *pharmacokinetics* of medications is critical to evaluating a new medication and implementing its use in clinical situations. A continuous infusion of any drug at a fixed rate will reach steady state in an exponential fashion. The half-life is the time it takes to achieve 50% of the steady-state concentration. Seventy-five percent of the steady-state concentration is achieved at 2 half-lives (60 minutes in our example). Ninety percent of the steady state is achieved by 3.3 half-lives (99 minutes in our example). Similarly, discontinuation of the drug will affect the concentration also in an exponential fashion.

26. **(E)** Insulin intake can lead to hypoglycemia, which is associated with appropriate pancreatic B-cell suppression and therefore low C peptide levels. Insulinomas are associated with hypoglycemia and C peptide levels. Glucagonomas, somatostatinomas, and Cushing syndrome are all associated with hyperglycemia.

27. **(D)**   Human placental lactogen is similar in structure to growth hormone. It causes insulin resistance, mobilization of free fatty acids, and increased insulin secretion. It is produced by the placenta and is detectable in serum at about 4 weeks' gestation.

28. **(E)**   When both members of a couple have a 1 in 30 chance, there is a $1/30 \times 1/30$ ($1/900$) chance that both will be carriers.

29. **(E)**   The malignant type of acanthosis nigricans may either precede, accompany, or follow the onset of internal cancer. Most cases are associated with adenocarcinoma of the stomach.

30. **(A)**   Calcium pyrophosphate dihydrate (CPPD) deposition in joint spaces can be asymptomatic but can present acutely as pseudogout. Gout most commonly affects the first metatarsophalangeal joint, whereas pseudogout affects the knee in 50%. Synovial fluid analysis can show inflammatory changes, with increases in the number of synovial leukocytes and neutrophils. Furthermore, CPPD crystals can be seen and are typically positively birefringent on polarized microscopy. Radiographically, chondrocalcinosis can be seen as an area of calcification in the fibrocartilage or hyaline. Pseudogout can be associated with a variety of metabolic derangements and disorders. Associations include hemochromatosis, hyperparathyroidism, hypothyroidism, hypophosphatasia, and hypomagnesemia. CPPD crystals and chondrocalcinosis are not features of rheumatoid arthritis. Gout is characterized by the presence of negatively birefringent monosodium urate crystals. Septic arthritis typically has even higher synovial leukocyte counts and is confirmed by Gram stain and cultures.

31. **(C)**   Muscle and cartilage tend to be radioresistant rather than sensitive. This is probably due to the fact that normal muscle and cartilage have a slow turnover rate and are thus affected less during cell cycling than cells in the bone marrow or gastrointestinal tract. The marrow and lymphoid system are the most radiosensitive tissues of the body. Sarcomas may develop after 20 years. One thousand rads can kill.

32. **(D)**   This is de Quervain's thyroiditis, which is self-limited. Only treatment with beta blocker is useful in the hyperthyroid phase. Methimazole and radioiodine are not effective. Surgery is not necessary.

33. **(A)**   The ulnar nerve innervates all of the intrinsic muscles of the hand except the lateral two lumbricales muscles, the opponens pollicis, the abductor pollicis brevis, and the flexor pollicis brevis. Chronic, severe compression of the ulnar nerve can lead to atrophy of most of the intrinsic muscles of the hand.

34. **(B)**   IgG is the only immunoglobulin capable of placental transfer.

35. **(A)**   Childhood dermtomyositis often presents with periorbital edema with a violaceous hue (heliotrope rash) and scaly erythematous plaques on the extremities. Muscle enzyme levels, particularly creatine kinase, may be elevated.

36. **(B)**   Wilms' tumor is the most common malignant neoplasm of the urinary tract in children. Ninety percent of Wilms' tumors present before age 7 years, with a peak between ages 3 and 4 years. Approximately 15 percent of Wilms' tumors have been associated congenital abnormalities of syndromes such as aniridia, hematoma, and hemihypertrophy. Beckwith-Wiedemann and WAGR syndromes (Wilms' tumor, aniridia, genital anomalies, and mental deficiency).

37. **(D)**   Stenosing tenosynovitis of the wrist is known as de Quervain's tendinitis. It is usually treated with rest of the hand, anti-inflammatory medication, steroid injection therapy, and, rarely, surgical release of the first dorsal compartment.

38. **(A)**   Koilocytosis (the development of a perinuclear clear space or halo) is associated with HPV infection. Multinucleated giant

cells are associated with the herpesvirus, and granuloma development can be associated with tuberculosis and syphilis. Plasma cell infiltration is seen in the endometrium with the diagnosis of chronic endometritis.

39. **(E)** Neuroblastoma is the second most common malignancy of infancy. Fifty percent of the cases present before age 2 years. Periorbital metastases are common, and retrobulbar soft tissue involvement causes periorbital edema and proptosis.

40. **(C)** A normal fasting glucose is less than 100 mg/dL. Impaired fasting glucose is a glucose between 100 and 126 mg/dL. Diabetes is defined by a fasting glucose of at least 126 mg/dL or above. Impaired glucose tolerance is a glucose of at least 200 mg/dL after an oral glucose load of 75 g.

41. **(C)** Regular Pap smear screening is a success story of early detection of precancerous changes in the cervix. Local treatment has been shown to be an effective way to prevent progression of preinvasive CIN. While false-negative readings can occur on Pap smears, the great majority of women diagnosed with invasive cervical cancer have not had screening in the past 7 years.

42. **(A)** The hormone pictured in this question is cortisol. It is synthesized in both the zona fasciculata and the zona reticularis. Cholesterol is converted to pregnenolone by P450scc (cholesterol side chain–cleaving enzyme). Pregnenolone is hydroxylated by P450c17 (17α-hydroxylase) to form 17α-hydroxypregnenolone. This hormone is converted to 17α-hydroxyprogesterone by 3α-hydroxysteroid dehydrogenase. P450c21 (21α-hydroxylase) then converts 17α-hydroxyprogesterone to 11-deoxycortisol, which is converted to cortisol by P450c11β (11β-hydroxylase). Cortisol cannot be synthesized by the zona glomerulosa because this zone does not contain P450c17.

43. **(D)** Tamoxifen, the oldest selective estrogen receptor modulator, is effective in the reduction of recurrence in selected breast cancers.

Bone-density testing in women on tamoxifen suggests that tamoxifen may in fact be protective against osteoporosis. There is no long-term evidence for or against the effect of tamoxifen on heart disease. Many studies have shown a two to three times increased risk for the development of endometrial cancer with the use of tamoxifen.

44. **(C)** The sensitivity and specificity of the tests are unique to the test and do not vary if the tests are identical. However, both the positive and the negative predictive value of the test can vary with the population. In the following table, the effect of increasing the prevalence increases the rate of true-positive tests (positive predictive value) and decreases the rate of true-negative tests (negative predictive value). Therefore, if the same test is being employed in two separate populations, the reason for a discrepancy in the rate of false-positive tests could be due to differences in the prevalence of the disease in the two separate populations. In particular, the higher the prevalence, the lower the rate of false-positive tests.

	Disease	No Disease
Test Positive	True Positive (a)	False Positive (b)
Test Negative	False Negative (c)	True Negative (d)
	(Prevalence)	

45. **(B)** Administration of leuprolide inhibits pulsatile secretion of GNRH by the hypothalamus and has the net effect of turning off ovarian function. While a GNRH agonist may be used in conjunction with ovulation-induction drugs to induce ovulation in infertile women, by itself it is an inhibitor of ovarian function and therefore causes amenorrhea.

46. **(B)** High-estrogen states such as pregnancy, oral contraceptives, or estrogen replacement therapy result in elevated levels of TBG. This protein carries about 70% of circulating thyroid hormones. In high-TBG states, total T_4 levels will be elevated, though free levels will be normal, reflecting a euthyroid state. A pituitary tumor secreting TSH would result in elevated free T_4 levels. Graves' disease is as-

sociated with a low TSH and elevated free T_4 levels. Iodine deficiency results in goiter and hypothyroidism. Thyroid carcinoma is nearly always associated with normal thyroid function tests.

47. **(D)** The normal ventilatory response is influenced by both the carbon dioxide and oxygen tension in the blood. However, hypoxemia has little influence on the ventilatory response until significant hypoxemia occurs (e.g., $PaO_2 < 60$ mmHg), whereas a strong relationship is seen with progressive hypocapnea. These relationships are depicted in Figure 2.5.

48. **(A)** The patient described likely has hepatopulmonary syndrome where intrapulmonary vascular dilatations in the setting of high cardiac outputs typical of cirrhotic patients behave as physiologic intrapulmonary shunts. Frank pulmonary arteriovenous malformations (AVMs) may also be evident. The orthodeoxia that was observed in this patient is thought to be due to enhanced shunting through AVMs that are primarily located in the lower lung zones where perfusion is greatest and is enhanced by being in the up-

right position. The lack of response to oxygen is typical of a shunt process, although the shunt can occur at any level, including intracardiac. Therefore, shunt is represented by the extreme of a low V/Q mismatch where effective ventilation is negligible or zero relative to the perfusion occurring through the shunt. Point A represents this extreme. Point C represents the other extreme where there is dead space (ventilation in an area of no perfusion). Hypoxemia due to V/Q mismatch is responsive to oxygen supplementation.

49. **(C)** A patient with obstructive sleep apnea will have closure of the upper airways during sleep. As the diaphragm contracts caudally to inspire, the abdominal contents are displaced, causing excursion of the abdominal band. However, because the upper airways are collapsed, the thorax cannot fill with air and symmetrically rise with the abdomen, leading to paradoxic out-of-phase movement of the thorax versus the abdomen. This finding is observed clinically as thoracoabdominal paradox and can also be seen in significant respiratory distress and diaphragmatic weakness. This paradox is seen in the tracing in C. Tracing B shows a normal in-

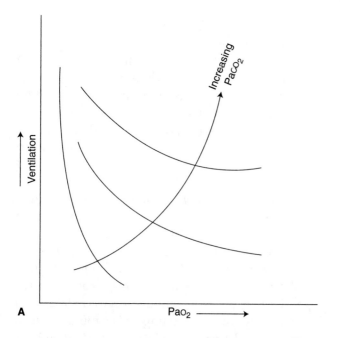
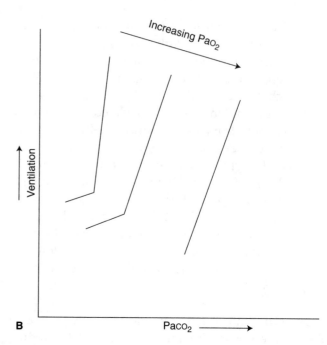

Figure 2.5 A and B

phase respiratory pattern, while A shows crescendo–descrescendo respiratory patterns but without paradox, as might be seen with central apneas. Tracing D likely shows a broken transducer on the abdominal band.

50. (A) Sebaceous glands are anatomically and functionally related to the hair follicle, and oversecretion of the sebaceous gland is one factor in the pathogenesis of acne.

Practice Test 3
Questions

DIRECTIONS (Questions 1 through 50): Each of the numbered items or incomplete statements in this section is followed by answers or by completions of the statement. Select the ONE lettered answer or completion that is BEST in each case.

1. A 60-year-old woman develops new left-sided headaches. She has had a diagnosis of polymyalgia rheumatica (PMR), and was successfully weaned off prednisone 3 months prior to presentation. Her laboratory studies reveal a mild anemia and a markedly elevated erythrocyte sedimentation rate (ESR) to 110 mm/hr. She has noticed some visual changes in her left eye. Which of the following is the next most appropriate step?

   (A) admit to hospital and initiate intravenous (IV) heparin for impending stroke
   (B) temporal artery biopsy
   (C) magnetic resonance imaging (MRI) of the head as an outpatient
   (D) immediate head computed tomographic (CT) scan
   (E) start nonsteroidal anti-inflammatory drugs (NSAIDs) and return in 3 days

2. A 58-year-old white man has undergone bilateral castration for management of his metastatic prostate cancer. Which of the following findings would be unlikely to be present on examination over time?

   (A) decreased facial hair
   (B) decreased libido
   (C) high voice
   (D) muscle weakness

   (E) elevated plasma follicle-stimulating hormone (FSH) levels

3. A 36-year-old man presents with refractory hypertension and is diagnosed with an aldosterone-secreting adrenal adenoma. Which of the following test results is consistent with the diagnosis?

   (A) hyperkalemia ✕
   (B) high serum renin
   (C) high serum angiotensin II
   (D) metabolic alkalosis
   (E) high serum cortisol

4. The eosinophilia commonly associated with human immunodeficiency virus (HIV) infection can be attributed to an increase in which cytokine?

   (A) interleukin-2 (IL-2)
   (B) interferon-alpha (IFN-α)
   (C) tumor necrosis factor-alpha (TNF-α)
   (D) IL-12
   (E) IL-5

5. An elderly man presents to the hospital and a presumptive diagnosis of Ogilvie's syndrome is made. Which of the following would be expected on abdominal imaging studies?

   (A) colonic and intestinal dilation and no free air
   (B) free intraperitoneal air
   (C) sigmoid or cecal volvulus
   (D) Meckel's diverticulum
   (E) cholelithiasis

6. A 22-year-old sexually active woman with a last menstrual period (LMP) 2 weeks ago presents to your office with a chief complaint of vaginal discharge, which is both copious and irritating. On speculum exam you see a foamy yellowish discharge coating the walls of her vagina, which look mildly inflamed. Her cervix also appears inflamed, and it occurs to you that the cervical surface resembles a strawberry. When you look at a wet mount of this discharge under the microscope you see motile organisms, which resemble those shown in Figure 3.1, along with normal-appearing epithelial cells and many white blood cells. What is the most likely diagnosis?

   (A) vulvovaginal candidiasis
   (B) trichomoniasis
   (C) recent intercourse
   (D) bacterial vaginosis
   (E) toxic shock syndrome

7. Which of the following disorders is caused by an RNA virus?

   (A) hand-foot-and-mouth disease
   (B) molluscum contagiosum
   (C) common warts
   (D) roseola
   (E) mononucleosis

8. A 24-year-old male patient presents with six episodes of this condition in the past year (see Figure 3.2). Which of the following medications is most likely to prevent future outbreaks?

   (A) acyclovir
   (B) itraconazole
   (C) erythromycin
   (D) methotrexate
   (E) diphenhydramine

9. The relapse rate of exacerbations in multiple sclerosis (MS) may be decreased by

   (A) beta-interferon IA
   (B) beta-interferon C
   (C) folic acid
   (D) methylprednisolone
   (E) dolobid

10. Which of the following antibodies is most commonly detected in patients with drug-induced systemic lupus erythematosus (SLE)?

   (A) double-stranded DNA (deoxyribonucleic acid)
   (B) antihistone
   (C) Ro(SSA)/La(SSB)
   (D) single-stranded DNA
   (E) anticentromere

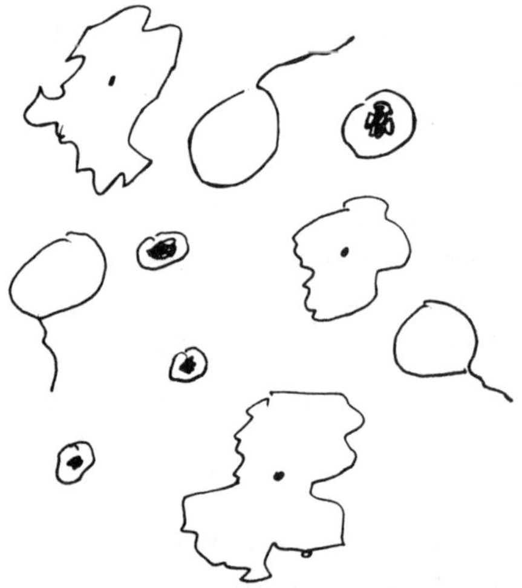

Figure 3.1

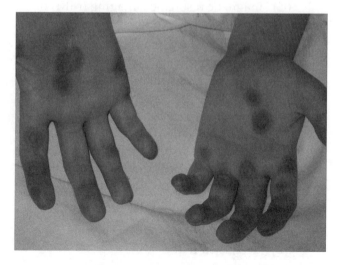

Figure 3.2

11. A 55-year-old African-American man presents with a 6-month history of low back pain and a hemoglobin of 9.8 g/dL. His peripheral smear is shown in Figure 3.3. What is the most likely diagnosis?

    (A) iron deficiency
    (B) anemia of chronic disease
    (C) spherocytosis
    (D) multiple myeloma
    (E) sickle cell trait

12. Lister's tubercle serves to allow the correct line of pull of which of the following tendons?

    (A) abductor pollicis brevis
    (B) extensor digiti minimi
    (C) extensor digitorum communis
    (D) extensor carpi radialis longus
    (E) extensor pollicis longus

13. The ulnar nerve innervates which of the following hand muscles?

    (A) adductor pollicis
    (B) abductor pollicis brevis
    (C) flexor pollicis brevis
    (D) opponens pollicis
    (E) radial two lumbricales

14. Regarding low-molecular-weight heparin (LMWH), which of the following statements is correct?

    (A) LMWH is given as an initial bolus dose followed by a continuous infusion.
    (B) The international normalized ratio (INR) is affected by LMWH.
    (C) LMWH inactivates factor X.
    (D) LMWH has a shorter half-life than does heparin.
    (E) LMWH affects the glycoprotein IIb/IIIa receptors.

15. Regarding hypertension in African-Americans, which of the following statements is correct?

    (A) Compared with whites, hypertension develops later in life.
    (B) The prevalence is lower in African-Americans than in whites.
    (C) Compared to whites, African-Americans receiving adequate treatment will have less overall decline in blood pressure.
    (D) Cardiovascular risk factors are more common in the African-American population.
    (E) Diuretics are of limited use in African-Americans.

16. A 54-year-old man with a long history of alcohol use and hepatitis C infection presents at the hospital with new onset of ascites. A paracentesis is performed, which shows a white blood cell count (WBC) of greater than 500/cc. A presumptive diagnosis of spontaneous bacterial peritonitis (SBP) is considered. What would be the most likely organism?

    (A) *Staphylococcus aureus*
    (B) *Streptococcus* sp.
    (C) *Pseudomonas* sp.
    (D) *Escherichia coli*
    (E) *Proteus* sp.

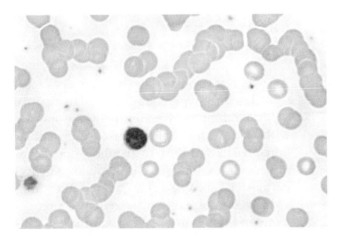

Figure 3.3

17. While being evaluated as a possible renal donor, a 40-year-old physician was noted to have bilateral multiple renal cysts. Small calcifications are present, and the kidneys are 22.1 × 12.8 × 14.5 and 20.5 × 12.0 × 15.1 cm. The potential donor's father died at age 52 of renal failure. The CT-scan evaluation of the abdomen showed cystic changes involving the spleen or pancreas. This patient's most likely diagnosis is

(A) tuberous sclerosis
(B) von Hippel–Lindau disease
(C) autosomal recessive polycystic disease
(D) acquired cystic disease
(E) autosomal dominant polycystic disease

18. A 34-year-old woman is seen because of rapidly accelerating hypertension. The patient has not been symptomatic. A renal arteriogram is done. The left renal arteriogram is normal; the right renal arteriogram shows a string of beads of the right renal artery. This woman's hypertension is due to

(A) renal artery arteriosclerosis
(B) intimal fibroplasias
(C) medial fibroplasias
(D) periadventitial fibroplasias
(E) renal arteriovenous (AV) fistula

19. Streptogranin antibiotics function by which of the following mechanisms?

(A) interfere with bacterial DNA synthesis
(B) inhibit bacterial protein synthesis
(C) inhibit bacterial mRNA synthesis
(D) inhibit bacterial adenosine triphosphatase (ATPase)
(E) nuclear cell damage

20. A newborn female has ambiguous genitalia. Blood studies reveal elevated dehydroepiandrosterone acetate sulfate (DHEAS) and 17α-hydroxyprogesterone levels. 11-Deoxycorticosterone levels are not elevated. Which is the most likely enzyme deficiency involved?

(A) P450c21 (21α-hydroxylase)
(B) P450c11β (11β-hydroxylase)
(C) P450scc (side-chain cleavage enzyme)
(D) 3α-hydroxysteroid dehydrogenase
(E) P450c17 (17α-hydroxylase)

21. A 56-year-old man was recently diagnosed with type 2 diabetes. After dietary changes have failed, you decide to give an agent to improve his glycemic control. He refuses to take the drug which can cause lactic acidosis. Which of the following drugs is he referring to?

(A) glyburide
(B) repaglinide
(C) pioglitazone
(D) metformin
(E) lisinopril

22. You are seeing an 18-year-old G1P0 patient in your office with a newly diagnosed pregnancy. The patient gives a history of regular, every-28-day menses until "a while ago." While the patient is uncertain of when her last menstrual period was, she has been feeling fetal movement for the last week or so. You are able to detect fetal heart tones with a handheld Doppler as well. Around how many weeks would you guess that the patient has been pregnant?

(A) 18
(B) 14
(C) 24
(D) 32
(E) 4–6

23. A 52-year-old nonsmoker complains of excessive daytime hypersomnolence. His spouse reports that he has severe disruptive snoring without any clear apneic episodes. Examination reveals an alert man who appears fatigued. On examination he is found to be hypertensive and severely obese. The lung sounds are normal, with excellent air movement and without wheezing. Cardiac auscultation reveals a mildly increased P2. A pulse oximetry reveals a saturation of 88%. An arterial blood gas is drawn and the results are listed in the following table. What is the likely cause of the patient's hypoxemia?

pH	7.38
Pco$_2$	60
Po$_2$	62
HCO$_3$	30

(A) alpha$_1$-antitrypsin deficiency

(B) chronic obstructive pulmonary disease

(C) idiopathic pulmonary fibrosis

(D) a chronic hypoventilatory syndrome

(E) chronic pulmonary embolism

24. An infant is born with annular erythematous plaques on the face and neck and is also noted to have bradycardia. Which diagnostic antibody test would be useful to confirm the diagnosis?

   (A) antiphospholipid
   (B) anti-Ro
   (C) antihistone
   (D) antiribonucleoprotein
   (E) anti-Smith

25. A 25-year-old woman is using a synthetic progestin for contraception. Which of the following adverse effects would be expected?

   (A) fluid loss
   (B) weight loss
   (C) thrombophlebitis
   (D) mania
   (E) improved lipid profile

Questions 26 through 30

Refer to the table below for questions 26 through 30.

	Cardiac Output	Systemic Vascular Resistance	Pulmonary Artery Occlusion Pressure
(A)	↓	↑	↓
(B)	↑	↓	↓ or No Change
(C)	↓	↑	↑
(D)	↑	↓	↓ or Normal

26. A 25-year-old man is brought to a trauma center following a severe motor vehicle accident. He is hypotensive and unresponsive. There is a large area of ecchymoses on his abdomen with gross distention. Intraperitoneal

hemorrhage is suspected. If a pulmonary artery catheter is utilized, which of the choices is likely to be found in this patient?

   (A) A
   (B) B
   (C) C
   (D) D
   (E) increased cardiac output only

27. A 71-year-old man has had multiple syncopal episodes prompting admission to the hospital. Shortly after arrival to the floor, the patient becomes acutely unresponsive and collapses on his bed. The patient has no pulse. The monitors reveal ventricular tachycardia. If a pulmonary artery catheter were to be in place, what would his measurements likely be from the above given choices?

   (A) A
   (B) B
   (C) C
   (D) D
   (E) increased cardiac output only

28. A 56-year-old man develops acute chest pain radiating to his left shoulder. He is also acutely dyspneic and found to be hypotensive. An electrocardiogram (ECG) shows 3-mm ST-segment elevations in the precordial leads. A chest x-ray reveals pulmonary edema. The patient is started on thrombolytic therapy for his acute myocardial infarction (MI). From the choices above, what is the likely reading if a pulmonary artery catheter is in place?

   (A) A
   (B) B
   (C) C
   (D) D
   (E) low systemic vascular resistance (SVR) only

29. A 68-year-old institutionalized woman is admitted to the hospital due to altered mental status. She is hypothermic and delirious. Her mental status deteriorates, with ensuing hypotension. A urine sample is grossly purulent, and blood cultures are drawn. What is the likely reading if a pulmonary artery catheter is in place?

   (A) A
   (B) B
   (C) C
   (D) D
   (E) low cardiac output and normal SVR

30. A 70-year-old man who lives alone is brought to the hospital after neighbors found him poorly responsive. The neighbors reported that he had been having chronic nausea, vomiting, and diarrhea for several weeks, but refused to seek medical care. He is hypotensive. Mucous membranes are dry, and his skin turgor is poor. What would his readings be if a pulmonary artery catheter were in place?

   (A) A
   (B) B
   (C) C
   (D) D
   (E) high cardiac output and high pulmonary artery occlusion pressure

31. In the event of disruption of the popliteal artery, which of the following vessels can provide some collateral flow to the lower leg?

   (A) femoral circumflex arteries
   (B) medial and lateral epiphyseal arteries
   (C) geniculate arteries
   (D) arcuate arteries
   (E) anterior and posterior tibial arteries

32. The presence of double-stranded DNA antibodies in SLE correlates best with involvement of which internal organ?

   (A) brain
   (B) kidney
   (C) liver

   (D) lung
   (E) heart

33. A 51-year-old man presents with palpitations. He has had intermittent diarrhea and weight loss as well. Examination reveals a mildly diaphoretic man with an irregularly irregular rhythm. (The heart rate is 110 beats per minute.) Neurologic exam reveals a mild proximal muscle weakness, diffusely increased reflexes, and a tremor. Neck exam also reveals a moderate-sized goiter. Suspecting hyperthyroidism, thyroid function tests were ordered. The sensitive thyroid-stimulating hormone (TSH) was at the upper end of normal, and the free thyroxine (free T_4) and triiodothyronine (T_3) were abnormally elevated. Of the choices given, what is the likely cause of this patient's hyperthyroidism?

   (A) the patient is not hyperthyroid as the s-TSH is a very sensitive test
   (B) surreptitious use of levothyroxine
   (C) Graves' disease
   (D) TSH-secreting pituitary adenoma
   (E) subacute thyroiditis

34. A 24-year-old woman with type 1 diabetes for 10 years is admitted to the hospital with diabetic ketoacidosis. She has severe metabolic acidosis due to high level of ketones. Which of the following is converted to ketone bodies when insulin is deficient?

   (A) glucose
   (B) fatty acids
   (C) amino acids
   (D) glycerol
   (E) cholesterol

35. Renin is largely produced from which of the following cells?

   (A) proximal nephron
   (B) distal tubule
   (C) juxtaglomerular cells
   (D) macula densa
   (E) cortex

36. A patient with advanced chronic obstructive pulmonary disease (COPD) is asked to blow out forcefully from full inspiration as fast and hard as she can, for as long as possible. Which of the graphs in Figure 3.4 is likely to reflect the patient's advanced COPD?

    (A) A
    (B) B
    (C) C
    (D) higher peak than A
    (E) lower levels than C

37. A 67-year-old woman has an ill-defined lung infiltrate described as a ground-glass opacity in the right upper lobe, which has slowly enlarged in the past year. The radiologist describes it to be an "alveolar" process. She has never smoked, and has recently noted some coughing and clear sputum production. Which of the following is likely?

    (A) squamous cell carcinoma
    (B) pneumonia
    (C) metastatic breast cancer

    (D) bronchioloalveolar cell carcinoma
    (E) small cell carcinoma

38. A 50-year-old man with a history of laryngeal carcinoma presents with increasing dyspnea. Stridor is evident, and the patient is in significant respiratory distress with visible accessory muscle use. A helium–oxygen mixture is applied to the patient in an attempt decrease the work of breathing while awaiting emergent ear, nose, and throat (ENT) assessment. What is the mechanism in which the helium–oxygen mixture might be able to alleviate some of the patient's work of breathing?

    (A) Helium lowers the Reynolds number.
    (B) The FiO_2 delivered can be higher in helium–oxygen mixtures.
    (C) Carbon dioxide is washed out more easily with helium mixtures.
    (D) Helium has bronchodilatory properties.
    (E) Alteration of voice and vocal cords.

39. Which of the following bacteria is the most common cause of septic arthritis in young adults?

    (A) *Chlamydia pneumoniae*
    (B) *Staphylococcus aureus*
    (C) *Vibrio parahaemolyticus*
    (D) *Neisseria gonorrhoeae*
    (E) *E. coli*

40. Most of the following are common causes of third-trimester vaginal bleeding. Which condition is often diagnosed in the first or early second trimester?

    (A) placenta previa
    (B) placental abruption
    (C) bloody show
    (D) ectopic pregnancy
    (E) abruptio placenta

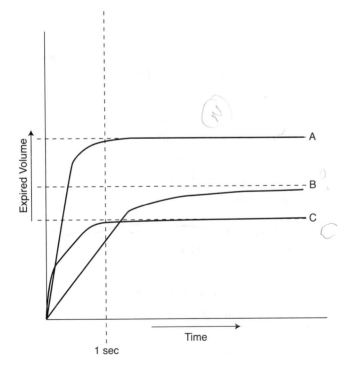

Figure 3.4

41. At which of the labeled sites of the pituitary gland shown in Figure 3-5 does synthesis of pro-opiomelanocortin occur?

    (A) A
    (B) B
    (C) C
    (D) D
    (E) E

Questions 42 through 45

42. A 64-year-old man with type 2 diabetes for 15 years is admitted to the hospital with hyperosmolar coma. On admission, his plasma glucose is 900 mg/dL. Which of the following treatments should be given first?

    (A) insulin infusion
    (B) half normal saline
    (C) normal saline
    (D) 5% dextrose
    (E) subcutaneous insulin

43. Which of the following ovarian conditions is most likely to be associated with hirsutism?

    (A) struma varii
    (B) mature ovarian teratoma
    (C) polycystic ovarian disease (PCO)
    (D) endometrioma
    (E) mucinous cystadenoma

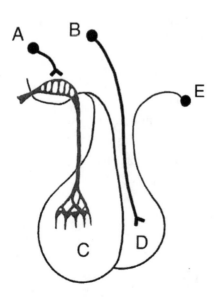

Figure 3.5

44. A patient presents with the "worst headache of her life." In the emergency department (ED), the patient has weakness of right eye muscles in all directions except abduction and inward torsion and has ptosis and mydriasis. A lumbar puncture reveals gross blood. An aneurysm is suspected. On which artery is the aneurysm likely to be located?

    (A) posterior communicating
    (B) anterior communicating
    (C) posterior inferior cerebellar (PICA)
    (D) posterior cerebral
    (E) middle cerebral

45. Which of the following refers to a painful sensation to a nonpainful stimulus?

    (A) dysesthesia
    (B) hyperpathia
    (C) hyperalgesia
    (D) parasthesia
    (E) allodynia

46. A 46-year-old man is brought by the police to the ED for confusion. He is disheveled and appears malnourished. There is a strong smell of alcohol. On his neurologic examination he is ataxic and is noted to have nystagmus and ophthalmoplegia. What is the most likely cause of this patient's neurologic findings?

    (A) vitamin A deficiency
    (B) vitamin A toxicity
    (C) vitamin B_{12} deficiency
    (D) vitamin C deficiency
    (E) thiamine deficiency

47. Which antibody is most strongly associated with photosensitivity?

    (A) Ro(SSA)
    (B) single-stranded DNA
    (C) double-stranded DNA
    (D) antihistone
    (E) anti-RNP

48. Most of the following medications used for stroke prophylaxis exhibit an antiplatelet effect. Which one affects the clotting cascade?

    (A) warfarin
    (B) aspirin
    (C) ticlopidine
    (D) clopidogrel
    (E) dipyridamole

49. A healthy 72-year-old woman presents with a painful vesicular rash in a bandlike distribution over her right lower abdomen. A Tzanck smear performed in the office demonstrates multinucleated giant cells. Which of the following is a varicella-zoster virus?

    (A) double-stranded DNA virus
    (B) parvovirus
    (C) poxvirus
    (D) single-stranded RNA virus
    (E) retrovirus

50. A 36-year-old woman is referred for further evaluation of porphyria. Preliminary laboratory evaluation reveals normal stool porphyrins. What is the most likely type of porphyria?

    (A) acute intermittent porphyria
    (B) erythropoietic porphyria
    (C) erythropoietic protoporphyria
    (D) porphyria cutanea tarda
    (E) variegate porphyria

Answers and Explanations

1. **(B)** This elderly woman has a new headache associated with some visual decline. This clinical picture and her prior history of having PMR strongly suggests the possibility of giant cell arteritis (GCA or temporal arteritis). Fifteen percent of patients with PMR will develop GCA, and half of those with GCA will have PMR. Steroids should be started immediately if the diagnostic test of choice (temporal artery biopsy) can not be done immediately. This is particularly important since this patient already has developed ocular symptoms that could result in permanent loss of vision. Studies have demonstrated that initiating steroids will not interfere with obtaining a pathologic diagnosis even after at least 2 weeks of therapy.

2. **(C)** Bilateral castration results in a marked reduction in circulating androgen levels. This condition is frequently associated with decreased facial hair, muscle weakness, poor energy, and decreased libido as well as impotence over time. FSH levels will be high due to lack of feedback inhibition by testosterone. At puberty, testosterone is responsible for laryngeal development and voice deepening. However, this effect is permanent, and in an adult hypogonadal male, the voice will remain deep.

3. **(D)** Aldosterone-secreting adenomas originate in the zona glomerulosa layer of the adrenal cortex. Excess levels of aldosterone and its precursors are secreted by this tumor and will inhibit renin and angiotensin II secretion. Aldosterone stimulates the renal secretion of potassium and hydrogen ions, and an excess of the hormone will be associated with hypokalemia and metabolic alkalosis. Cortisol cannot be produced by the zona glomerulosa, and therefore levels will not be elevated.

4. **(E)** IL-5 is responsible for eosinophil differentiation. In HIV infection the TH_2 phenotype predominates with resultant IL-4, IL-5, and IL-10 production.

5. **(A)** Acute colonic pseudo-obstruction is more common in elderly men over the age of 60 and generally presents with nausea, vomiting, and abdominal pain. Pathophysiologically, the condition results from a lack of colonic motility. Plain and upright abdominal radiographs will demonstrate a markedly dilated colon, extending from the cecum to the sigmoid colon. Free intraperitoneal air would suggest the presence of a perforation of the colon in this setting. A colonoscopy or gentle Hypaque (water soluble) enema is useful in not only confirming the diagnosis but also as a potential treatment strategy. There is lack of either a cecal or sigmoid volvulus in patients with this syndrome.

6. **(B)** All of the signs and symptoms and findings are associated with *Trichomonas*. While spermatozoa appear motile under the microscope, they are of a smaller size and different shape from trichomonads. Bacterial vaginosis causes a fishy vaginal odor, and "clue cells"—epithelial cells coated with bacteria—are seen on wet mount and no WBCs are seen.

7. **(A)** Hand-foot-and-mouth disease is caused by coxsackievirus, an NA virus. All of the other entities are caused by a DNA virus.

8. **(A)** Herpesvirus infections may cause recurrent outbreaks of erythema multiforme, depicted here as annular plaques on the palms. The treatment of choice in this setting is an antiviral medication such as acyclovir.

9. **(A)** Intravenous methylprednisolone at a dose of 1 g daily for 3 to 5 days may decrease severity and shorten the duration of an MS attack but does not affect relapse rate. Mitoxantrone also has affect on the progressive form of MS but has the potential for serious cardiotoxicity. Beta-interferon IA has also been shown to decrease long-term disability and prevent some of the cognitive symptoms associated with MS. Glatiramer acetate and mitoxantrone may also be of value.

10. **(B)** Ninety percent of patients with drug-induced SLE have antihistone antibodies.

11. **(D)** This is a classic illustration of rouleaux formation and is very consistent with this clinical history. More than 80% of patients have monoclonal immunoglobulin in their serum, which causes rouleaux formation. Fifteen percent will have only hypogammaglobulinemia and monoclonal light chains in the urine. Rouleaux formation may also be due to polyclonal hypergammaglobulinemia or hyperfibrinogenemia. However, in this patient with low back pain, this is highly suggestive of myeloma.

12. **(E)** The extensor pollicis longus tendon runs along the ulnar side of Lister's tubercle, then diagonally across the wrist. This allows the tendon to function as a true extensor of the thumb.

13. **(A)** The adductor pollicis and all other intrinsics of the hand are innervated by the ulnar nerve. The radial nerve is sensory only in the hand.

14. **(C)** LMWH is administered as a twice-daily subcutaneous injection and does not require monitoring the partial thromboplastin time (PTT) or INR. It inactivates factor X. In patients with renal dysfunction, anti–factor X can be monitored and the drug should be used only with caution since it is renally cleared. LMWH is not a glycoprotein IIb/IIIa receptor antagonist.

15. **(D)** The prevalence of hypertension in African-Americans is among the highest in the world. Hypertension develops at earlier ages, and there are a greater number with stage 3 hypertension. Complications of hypertension are higher in African-Americans. On adequate therapy, hypertension responds similarly. There is a higher prevalence of cardiovascular risk factors such as obesity, smoking, and type 2 diabetes in African-Americans. In both African-Americans and whites, diuretics have been proven to reduce morbidity and mortality from hypertension. It should be given as the initial drug of choice in the absence of a specific contraindication.

16. **(D)** SBP generally occurs in patients with chronic liver disease and cirrhosis and by definition impies that there is an ascitic fluid infection without an evident intra-abdominal surgically treatable source. The diagnosis is established by the use of paracentesis in which there is a positive ascitic fluid bacterial culture and an elevated ascitic fluid.

17. **(E)** Renal cysts are encountered in several hereditary syndromes. The most common cystic kidney disease is adult polycystic disease (APCD). The inheritance is autosomal dominant. Clinical features are a positive family history, flank masses, hypertension, and azotemia. The age at onset of symptoms ranges from 10 to more than 90 years of age. The median age of death for APCD is 50 years.

18. **(C)** Medical fibroplasia produces a "string of beads" appearance at renal arteriography. This is the most common of the fibrous arterial lesions, constituting 75% to 80% of the total.

19. **(B)** Streptogranin antibiotics are composed of two chemically distinct compounds. These

synergistically act to inhibit protein synthesis. They have a broad spectrum of activity against gram-negative bacteria and are effective against multidrug-resistant organisms.

20. **(A)** Deficiency of P450c21 results in accumulation of 17α-hydroxyprogesterone and an increase in its conversion to adrenal androgens such as DHEA, DHEAS, and androstenedione. Deficiency of P450c11β leads to accumulation of 11-deoxycorticosterone. 3α-Hydroxysteroid dehydrogenase deficiency results in decreased 17α-hydroxyprogesterone levels. P450c17 deficiency is associated with decreased 17α-hydroxyprogesterone levels and decreased adrenal androgen production.

21. **(D)** Metformin can lead to lactic acidosis, mainly in patients who have renal failure, heart failure, liver disease, or severe infections.

22. **(A)** At around 20 weeks' gestation (counting from the last menstrual period, and therefore about 18 weeks from conception), the uterine fundus reaches the height of the umbilicus. Quickening, or maternal perception of fetal movement, generally occurs at 16 to 18 weeks' gestation in women having their first babies. Fetal heart tones are generally easily heard by Doppler at 20 weeks' gestation.

23. **(D)** The patient is hypoxemic, as suggested by the reduced saturation and arterial oxygen tension. The P_{CO_2} is elevated but the pH is within normal, suggesting that the abnormalities are chronic and that the patient is well compensated. The cause of the hypoxemia is evident when the alveolar-to-arterial oxygen gradient (A-a gradient) is calculated. If this is done, the A-a gradient is normal, suggesting that the hypoxemia can be attributed to the elevation in the P_{CO_2}. The isolated elevation of the P_{CO_2} is the setting of a normal A-a gradient suggests a chronic hypoventilatory syndrome. The clinical picture described is best compatible with the obesity–hypoventilatory syndrome, which is strongly associated with

obstructive sleep apnea. Although all the other choices could cause hypoxemia, the A-a gradient would have been expected to be abnormal.

24. **(B)** Neonatal lupus erythematosus is characterized by congenital heart block or annular papulosquamous skin lesions or both. Anti-Ro is a diagnostic marker for neonatal lupus erythematosus. The condition arises as a result of passive transfer of maternal antibodies.

25. **(C)** Progestins stimulate appetite and cause weight gain. They may also cause fluid retention, thrombophlebitis and deep venous thrombosis, decreased high-density lipoprotein (HDL) cholesterol, and depression.

26–30. **(26-A, 27-C, 28-C, 29-D, 30-A)** *Shock* is characterized by a state in which tissue perfusion is significantly reduced. There are several types of shock, but the three general classes most commonly referred to are hypovolemic, cardiogenic, and distributive shock. Hypovolemic shock can arise from hemorrhage or fluid losses. Specific causes include trauma, vomiting, diarrhea, burns, insensible losses, gastrointestinal (GI) bleeding, or aortic rupture. In these states, the preload is reduced, and on a pulmonary artery catheter, the preload to the left ventricle can be estimated by the pulmonary artery occlusion (or wedge) pressure (PAOP). Therefore, in cases of hypovolemic shock, the PAOP should be reduced with a concomitant drop in the cardiac output. The systemic vascular resistance (SVR) is increased in response to the hypovolemia and fall in cardiac output.

In cardiogenic shock, the primary problem is that of pump failure. This can be due to valvular disease, malignant arrhythmias, or ventricular failure (e.g., MI, congestive heart failure). In these situations, the cardiac output measurements will be low, and because of poor forward flow, the PAOP will increase. The SVR also increases in response to the hypotension. Finally, distributive shock refers to a state of effective hypovolemia in the absence of real volume depletion. Examples include septic shock, toxic shock syndromes, neurogenic shock (e.g., spinal cord injury, epidural anesthesia), anaphylaxis, and addisonian crisis. The primary perturbation in distributive shock is a fall in the SVR. Early on (preshock), there may be a compensatory hyperdynamic response with an increase in the cardiac output, but with progression the cardiac output will fall.

31. **(C)** Four geniculate arteries (two superior and two inferior) supply the anterior knee and can provide minimal collateral flow to the lower leg when the popliteal artery is disrupted or blocked.

32. **(B)** Anti-ds DNA is associated with nephritis and clinical activity.

33. **(D)** The patient described is clinically hyperthyroid. This is compatible with the elevated free T_4 and T_3. However, the s-TSH is not suppressed as it should be if a patient had primary hyperthyroidism. The most likely reason is that the patient has secondary hyperthyroidism, which is reflected by the inappropriately normal s-TSH, although frequently they are elevated as well. This combination of a hyperthyroid patient with elevation in T_4 and T_3, and a normal or elevated s-TSH is not characteristic of the other choices. The next best step in the evaluation of this patient is an MRI to look for a TSH-secreting pituitary adenoma.

34. **(B)** When insulin is deficient, counterregulatory hormones (glucagons, epinephrine, cortisol, and growth hormone) rise, causing increased lipolysis and elevated fatty acids. The fatty acids are converted to ketone bodies in the liver.

35. **(C)** The major source of active renin is the juxtaglomerular apparatus in the kidney. The major cells are the juxtaglomerular cells and rarely from macula densa cells or the distal convoluted tubule.

36. **(b)** A patient with COPD has ventilatory limitation with forced expiration due to poor elastic recoil and increased resistance to airflow. On forced rapid exhalation from full inspiration (forced vital capacity maneuver), the flow is diminished (as represented by the slope of the curve), and often patients with advanced COPD can have a very prolonged expiratory phase before plateauing at their forced vital capacity (FVC). Because of the airflow resistance and loss of elastic recoil, the expired volume in the first second (FEV_1) is reduced when compared to the FVC in COPD and is graphically represented in patient B. Restrictive diseases such as pulmonary fibrosis also have a reduced FVC but there is no limitation to airflow, and patients are able to achieve their reduced FVC rapidly as in tracing C. The FEV_1 approximates the FVC in this case. Tracing A shows a more normal tracing with a higher FVC and an FEV_1 that approaches this.

37. **(D)** Ground-glass opacities defined by preservation of normal lung architecture through a hazy infiltrate radiographically is most suggestive of an "alveolar" process. Occasionally, fine microscopic interstitial processes can appear as ground-glass lesions. Although alveolar processes typically reflect edema, hemorrhage, or pneumonia where the alveoli is flooded with fluid or cells, malignanices can also present in such a fashion, including bronchioloalveolar cell carcinoma (BAC) in which the malignant cells grows along the alveolar walls without significant distortion of the underlying lung architecture. This malignancy can be slow growing and is least associated with smoking. The lack of a "solid" appearance as is typical of the other malignancies listed should therefore not exclude the possibility of a malignancy. The persistence of the infiltrate and the lack of typical infectious symptoms exclude pneumonia.

38. **(A)** The Reynolds number is proportional to the gas density, air flow, and radius of the

airway, and inversely proportional to the gas viscosity. The higher the Reynolds number, the more turbulent the air flow. Laminar air flow as occurs in the small distal airways is independent of the density of gas, but in the central airways or at sites of obstruction, as in this patient, the air flow is turbulent and dependent on the gas density. The air flow resistance across the obstruction in this patient is the primary reason for the increased work of breathing. Since helium is less dense than oxygen or ambient air, air flow across the obstruction can be improved, leading to reduced work of breathing. The other choices are incorrect and do not address the primary reason for the increase in patient's work of breathing.

39. **(D)** *Neisseria gonorrhoeae* is four times more common in women than in men. Joint aspiration yields a WBC of 30,000 to 100,000. Cervical or urethral cultures are positive most of the time. Initial treatment is usually with a beta-lactamase-resistant cephalosporin given intravenously.

40. **(D)** Ectopic pregnancy is usually diagnosed in the first or early second trimester of pregnancy. All of the other conditions usually present with third-trimester bleeding.

41. **(C)** Pro-opiomelanocortin is secreted by corticotroph cells in the anterior pituitary. This molecule is a precursor to corticotropin (ACTH) and melanocyte-stimulating hormone. *A* represents a hypothalamic neurosecretory neuron, *B* the paraventricular and supraoptic nuclei of the hypothalamus, and *D* the posterior pituitary.

42. **(C)** Fluids should be given prior to insulin; otherwise, shock may result (due to entry of glucose and water inside the cells, leading to more volume depletion). Normal saline is always given first, followed by half normal when volemic status has been somewhat restored; 5% dextrose is added when plasma glucose is lowered to around 250 mg/dL.

43. **(C)** PCOD is the most common cause of hirsutism in women. While mature teratomas can contain hair, they are not associated with male-pattern external hair as characterizes hirsutism. Struma ovarii describes an ovarian neoplasm formed by ectopic thyroid tissue. Endometriomas and mucinous cystadenomas are benign causes of ovarian enlargement and are not associated with hirsutism.

44. **(A)** This patient has a pupil-involving third cranial nerve palsy. Involvement of the pupillary fibers suggests extrinsic compression of the nerve. The posterior communicating artery sits in close proximity to the nerve as it exits the midbrain. The middle cerebral and anterior communicating arteries are two other likely sites for a cerebral aneurysm.

45. **(E)** Allodynia is commonly found during examination of a patient with neuropathic pain along with hyperpathia (pain produced with repetitive stimulus) and hyperalgesia (excess pain from a painful stimulus). Dysesthesia may be painful but is spontaneous, not evoked by stimulus. Paresthesia is a non-painful sensation.

46. **(E)** The triad of ataxia, nystagmus, and ophthalmoplegia is referred to as Wernicke's encephalopathy. It results from thiamine deficiency and occurs usually in chronic alcoholics. This syndrome is treatable, and administration of thiamine should be initiated intravenously, particularly before any administration of dextrose-containing solutions. Korsakoff's psychosis presents with impaired short-term memory and confabulation and is part of the spectrum of Wernicke-Korsakoff syndrome (cerebral beriberi). Korsakoff's psychosis is less responsive to treatment. Thiamine deficiency can also cause peripheral neuropathy (dry beriberi), and high-output cardiac failure (wet beriberi).

47. **(A)** Ro(SSA) antibodies are strongly associated with photosensitivity.

48. (A) Warfarin exerts its effect at the clotting cascade. Aspirin may also act as a prostaglandin inhibitor in preventing stroke.

49. (A) Varicella-zoster virus is a double-stranded DNA virus, which causes varicella and herpes zoster. Parvovirus and poxvirus are other double-stranded DNA viruses. Human immunodeficiency virus (HIV) is an example of a retrovirus.

50. (A) Normal stool porphyrins are most likely to occur in acute intermittent porphyria. The enzymatic deficiency in this disease is early in the heme biosynthetic pathway, resulting in overproduction of water-soluble precursors. All of the other porphyrias listed have associated stool findings.

Practice Test 4
Questions

DIRECTIONS (Questions 1 through 50): Each of the numbered items or incomplete statements in this section is followed by answers or by completions of the statement. Select the ONE lettered answer or completion that is BEST in each case.

1. A 45-year-old woman is diagnosed with thyroid cancer and undergoes a total thyroidectomy. Which of the following is a complication of this surgery?

    (A) hyperthyroidism
    (B) hypercalcemia
    (C) damage to the recurrent laryngeal nerve and tetany
    (D) hypoglycemia
    (E) hypertension

2. An 80-year-old man presents with early satiety and a spleen measuring 10 cm below the left costal margin. A complete blood count (CBC) is obtained, with a hemoglobin of 11 g/dL, a white blood cell count (WBC) of 86,000/μL, and a platelet count of 560,000/μL. Ultrasound confirms the presence of an enlarged spleen. Which of the following is the most likely diagnosis?

    (A) chronic lymphocytic leukemia (CLL)
    (B) hereditary spherocytosis
    (C) lupus
    (D) chronic myelogenous leukemia (CML)
    (E) mononucleosis

3. Which of the following is reported to induce pseudoporphyria?

    (A) erythromycin
    (B) methotrexate
    (C) 8-methoxypsoralen
    (D) naproxen
    (E) ethanol

4. Pseudomembraneous colitis is associated with which of the following organisms?

    (A) *Campylobacter* sp.
    (B) *Escherichia coli*
    (C) *Clostridium difficile*
    (D) *Helicobacter pylori*
    (E) *Pseudomonas* sp.

5. Which of the following antibiotics is appropriate for treating an elderly patient diagnosed with pseudomembranous colitis?

    (A) ampicillin
    (B) ampicillin plus gentamicin
    (C) erythromycin
    (D) vancomycin or metronidazole
    (E) penicillin

6. A severely malnourished indigent patient is admitted to the hospital with ecchymoses. In addition to the ecchymoses, she has perifollicular petechiae, bleeding gums, and hyperkeratosis. What is the likely cause of the patient's symptoms and signs?

    (A) vitamin A deficiency
    (B) vitamin A toxicity
    (C) vitamin B_{12} deficiency
    (D) vitamin C deficiency
    (E) vitamin K deficiency

7. A 30-year-old woman with anemia presents with thrombocytopenia and right hemiparesis. She is found to have a hemoglobin of 8.8, a platelet count of 24,000/μL, and a creatinine (Cr) of 2.2. A peripheral smear is obtained (Figure 4.1). What is the most likely diagnosis?

(A) spherocytosis
(B) immune thrombocytopenic purpura
(C) thrombotic thrombocytopenic purpura (TTP)
(D) vitamin B$_{12}$ deficiency
(E) malaria

8. A 66-year-old woman with end-stage renal disease presents with shaking, sweating, and dizziness and is found to be hypoglycemic. Which of the following would she exhibit?

(A) decreased glucagon release from pancreatic islet cells
(B) decreased gluconeogenesis
(C) pituitary corticotropin (ACTH) inhibition
(D) decreased adipocyte lipolysis
(E) increased parasympathetic nervous system activity

9. One of your friends from college recently has found out that she is pregnant after trying to conceive for about 6 months. She has always had every-28-day menses and knows that the first day of her last menstrual period (LMP) was 8/15/04. What is her estimated date of delivery (EDD)?

(A) 5/22/04
(B) 4/22/05
(C) 6/22/05
(D) 5/15/05
(E) 5/22/05

10. The pathologic finding shown in Figure 4.2 is found in which of the following?

(A) Alzheimer's disease
(B) Parkinson's disease
(C) Wilson's disease
(D) Pick's disease
(E) Huntington's chorea

11. Which of the following muscle groups should be strengthened following a tear of the anterior cruciate ligament (ACL)?

(A) gastrocnemius/soleus
(B) quadriceps
(C) hamstrings
(D) adductor magnus/adductor longus
(E) gluteus maximus

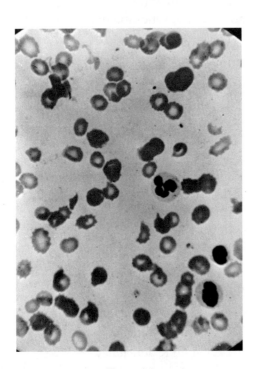

Figure 4.1

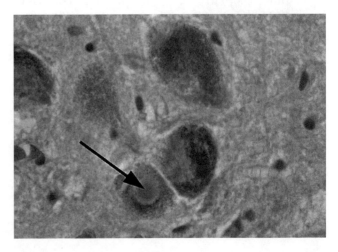

Figure 4.2

12. The PR interval on an electrocardiogram (ECG) is comprised of which of the following?

    (A) the time it takes for electricity to be generated by the sinus node and travel through the atrium
    (B) the time it takes for the ventricles to depolarize completely
    (C) the time it takes for the impulse to travel through the atrium, the atrioventricular (AV) node, and the His bundle
    (D) the time required to complete systole
    (E) the time required for diastolic activation

13. During an abdominal ultrasonographic examination for abdominal/flank pain and fever, a 45-year-old hypertensive man with a family history of renal failure was noted to have bilaterally enlarged cystic kidneys an hepatic and pancreatic cysts. He also complained of marked dysuria. Urine cultures were obtained, and he was admitted with a presumptive diagnosis of pyelonephritis. While awaiting culture results, the best initial antibiotic is which of the following?

    (A) gentamicin
    (B) ampicillin
    (C) cephalexin
    (D) trimethoprim
    (E) nitrofurantoin

14. You are investigating the cause of recurrent hypoglycemia in a 35-year-old man. At the time, the plasma glucose is 30 mg/dL with symptoms, the insulin level is high, but the C peptide level is low. Which of the following is causing the patient's hypoglycemia?

    (A) insulinoma
    (B) sulfonylurea use
    (C) adrenal insufficiency
    (D) insulin use
    (E) growth hormone deficiency

15. A 34-year-old woman is diagnosed with insulinoma. She also has a history of prolactinoma and primary hyperparathyroidism. She has

    (A) multiple endocrine neoplasia type 1 (MEN 1)
    (B) MEN 2A
    (C) MEN 2B
    (D) MEN 3
    (E) MEN 4

16. Krukenberg's tumors are a certain type of tumor that comes from another primary site and metastasizes to the ovary. What cell type is seen when a Krukenberg's tumor is diagnosed?

    (A) Sertoli-Leydig cell
    (B) granulosa cells
    (C) signet cells
    (D) squamous cells
    (E) immature neural tissue

17. When a Krukenberg's tumor is found, what is the most common site of the primary cancer?

    (A) stomach
    (B) breast
    (C) colon
    (D) endometrium
    (E) thyroid

18. Which of the following is a risk factor for the development of low back problems?

    (A) aerobic exercise
    (B) gentle stretching
    (C) job dissatisfaction
    (D) prolonged walking
    (E) meditation

19. After 7 days of therapy with clindamycin for a *Bacteroides fragilis* pelvic infection, a 47-year-old man develops persistent bloody diarrhea, abdominal pain, and fever. A stool assay for *Clostridium difficile* is positive. In addition to discontinuing the clindamycin, the best management is

(A) opiates
(B) cefoxitin
(C) metronidazole
(D) chloramphenicol
(E) cholestyramine

20. A 30-year-old woman presents to you for a routine obstetric visit. She is 20 weeks pregnant. Which of the following hormonal conditions is present in this patient?

(A) Serum human chorionic gonadotropin (hCG) levels are increasing.
(B) Oophorectomy would result in a spontaneous abortion.
(C) Serum luteinizing hormone (LH) is elevated.
(D) Human placental lactogen (hPL) levels are increasing.
(E) Prolactin levels are peaking.

21. Which of the following properties are shared by glucagon and cortisol?

(A) They are steroid hormones.
(B) They are extensively bound by plasma proteins.
(C) They stimulate gluconeogenesis.
(D) They are inhibited by hypoglycemia.
(E) They stimulate glycogenolysis.

22. A 21-year-old woman presents with chronic low back pain, mild pancytopenia, splenomegaly, and x-rays with abnormalities of the vertebral bodies and pelvis. What is the most likely diagnosis?

(A) hereditary spherocytosis
(B) CML
(C) multiple myeloma
(D) CLL
(E) Gaucher's disease

23. A 51-year-old previously healthy white woman was admitted to a local hospital complaining of fatigue, weakness, lethargy, a 30-pound weight loss over a period of 1 month, and diffuse abdominal cramping pain without other gastrointestinal symptoms. On physical examination, the patient had a confused sensorium and appeared ill. Blood pressure is 200/120 mmHg, heart rate is 120 beats per minute, respirations are 20 per minute, and temperature is normal. No skin rash or arthritis is noted. Examination of the abdomen reveals hypoactive bowel sounds; diffuse tenderness without rebound, and hemoccult-positive stools. There is no evidence of hepatomegaly or splenomegaly and no adenopathy.

Laboratory Studies

Serum creatinine	2.5 mg/dL		Serum bilirubin	6.7 mg/dL
Hemoglobin	9.4 g/dL		Platelets	32,000/mm^3
Leukocyte count	11,000/mm^3		Rheumatoid factor	Positive (1:320)
Antinuclear antibodies	Negative			
Urinalysis	Protein 3+, > 100 RBCs/ hpf			

Chest radiography reveals patchy acinar and interstitial infiltrates. An abdominal radiograph reveals ileus. Abdominal and renal ultrasound are normal. Which of the following diagnostic studies should be done next?

(A) percutaneous liver biopsy
(B) mesenteric angiography
(C) serum cryoglobulin and/or cryocrit
(D) colonoscopy
(E) open liver biopsy

24. Regarding mitral valve prolapse (MVP), which of the following statements is correct?

(A) It is caused by protrusion of the mitral valve into the left atrium during diastole when the valve should be closed.
(B) It is an infrequent form of cardiac valvular abnormality.

(C) Patients with mitral valve prolapse may develop ventricular arrhythmias.

(D) MVP is caused by extra long chordae tethering the mitral valve.

(E) All patients with MVP should receive prophylactic antibiotics.

25. Routine ophthalmologic examination of a 16-year-old boy reveals a Lisch nodule. This ocular lesion is characteristic of

(A) tuberous sclerosis

(B) neurofibromatosis

(C) Marfan's syndrome

(D) Down's syndrome

(E) xeroderma pigmentosum

26. A 37-year-old white man with a 5-year history of ulcerative colitis now in remission presents to the emergency department (ED) with a 1-day history of severe right upper quadrant pain, nausea, vomiting, and fever. Physical examination reveals the patient to be in moderate distress, with a temperature of 38.4°C (101.2°F) and a normal blood pressure. Oral examination reveals no aphthous ulcerations. Conjunctival icterus is noted on eye examination. Examination of the abdomen reveals normal bowel sounds and right upper quadrant tenderness without rebound. There is no hepatomegaly noted, and a Murphy's sign is absent. The spleen is not palpable, and there is no adenopathy. Rectal examination is normal and hemoccult negative.

Laboratory Studies

Leukocyte count	16,000/mm^3; 80% neutrophils, 10% bands
Hemoglobin	14.4 g/dL
Electrolytes	Normal
Alkaline phosphatase	400 U/L
Aspartate transaminase (AST) and alanine transaminase (ALT)	Normal
Bilirubin, total	4 mg/dL

Chest and abdominal radiographs are normal. An abdominal ultrasound reveals a dilated common bile duct and intrahepatic ducts, but gallstones or common bile duct stones are absent. Which of the following statements is correct?

(A) A diagnosis of primary biliary cirrhosis should be excluded by liver biopsy.

(B) Gallstones are less likely to occur in patients with ulcerative colitis.

(C) Sclerosing cholangitis should be excluded in this patient by endoscopic retrograde cholangiopancreatography (ERCP) evaluation.

(D) HIDA (hepato-iminodiacetic acid) imaging has a low sensitivity for diagnosing acute cholecystitis.

(E) The patient may be discharged and monitored at home.

27. Which of the following agents would be expected to increase bowel motility?

(A) bethanecol

(B) morphine sulfate

(C) histamine 2 (H$_2$) receptor antagonists

(D) dopamine antagonists

(E) amoxicillin

28. The term *burst fracture* of the lumbar spine implies

(A) narrowing of the pedicles on an anteroposterior (AP) x-ray

(B) retropulsion of the posterior vertebral body

(C) undamaged vertebral body

(D) no neurologic impairment proportionate to the degree of canal compromise

(E) "blowout" fracture

29. Lumbar burst fractures are due to which of the following mechanisms?

(A) flexion

(B) extension

(C) rotation

(D) distraction

(E) axial loading

30. The sartorius muscle functions as a

    (A) hip flexor and knee flexor
    (B) hip extensor and knee flexor
    (C) hip adductor
    (D) knee extensor
    (E) hip abductor

31. Which of the following conditions becomes more common in women after menopause?

    (A) osteoporosis and macular degeneration
    (B) viral diseases
    (C) breast cysts
    (D) sunburn
    (E) allergies

32. A patient with bronchogenic lung cancer has a large pleural effusion in association with atelectasis of the left lower lobe. Thoracentesis is unlikely to reexpand the lung in a situation where the cause of the pleural effusion is

    (A) due to pleural metastases
    (B) due to a complicated parapneumonic effusion
    (C) secondary to a chylothorax from lymphatic disruption from the tumor
    (D) secondary to an endobronchial lesion
    (E) unknown causes

33. A 72-year-old man presents with a fluctuant parotid mass that he has ignored for the past 10 years. He states there has been little growth over those 10 years, with no pain, headaches, paralysis, weight loss, xerostomia, and lymphadenopathy. What is the most likely diagnosis?

    (A) mucoepidermoid carcinoma
    (B) papillary cystadenoma
    (C) adenoid cystic carcinoma
    (D) lymphoma
    (E) pleomorphic adenoma

34. Which of the following agents may produce peripheral neuropathy?

    (A) lead and acrylamide
    (B) vitamin C (high dose)
    (C) benzene
    (D) propane
    (E) erythromycin

35. A 50-year-old man presents with proximal muscle weakness and pain. His creatine phosphokinase (CPK) is elevated at 8000 (normal < 200). An electromyogram (EMG) reveals myopathic motor units. A muscle biopsy of the right quadriceps reveals regenerating and degenerating muscle cells, perifascicular muscle cell atrophy, lymphocytic inflammatory cells, and perivascular inflammation. What diagnosis does the muscle pathology suggest?

    (A) polymyositis
    (B) dermatomyositis
    (C) inclusion body myositis
    (D) viral myositis
    (E) vasculitis

36. Donepezil, galantamine, and rivastigmine have been shown to be beneficial in the treatment of patients with Alzheimer's disease. What is their mechanism of action?

    (A) anticholinergic
    (B) cholinesterase inhibitor
    (C) serotonin reuptake inhibitor
    (D) serotonin and norepinephrine reuptake inhibitor
    (E) choline acetyltransferase blocker

37. Regarding coronary revascularization in patients with unstable angina or non-ST-segment elevation myocardial infarction (MI), which of the following statements is true?

    (A) Percutaneous coronary intervention (PCI) should be performed in patients with left main stenosis.
    (B) PCI or coronary artery bypass grafting (CABG) is not indicated in patients with one- or two-vessel coronary disease in the absence of proximal left anterior descending disease.
    (C) Repeat CABG should not be undertaken in patients with prior bypass grafting.
    (D) PCI should not be done in patients with multivessel disease.
    (E) CABG remains experimental in treating multivessel disease.

38. Which alpha₁-antitrypsin phenotype is a risk factor for severe emphysema but never liver disease?

    (A) null-null
    (B) MM
    (C) SZ
    (D) MZ
    (E) ZZ

39. The temperature chart in Figure 4.3 indicates probable

    (A) anovulation
    (B) luteal-phase defect
    (C) pregnancy
    (D) fever of unknown origin (FUO)
    (E) malaria

40. Which of the following statements is true concerning oropharyngeal cancers?

    (A) They are generally adenocarcinomas.
    (B) They do not spread locally to the appropriate cervical lymph nodes.
    (C) They can be multifocal and are generally caused by smoking.
    (D) They are generally due to ingesting cold beverages.
    (E) Early-stage tumors are rarely curable with surgery alone.

41. Which of the following may be associated with MVP?

    (A) arrhythmia and sudden death in up to 1.9% of patients
    (B) no complications
    (C) left arm pain and diaphoresis
    (D) early systolic click
    (E) inherited as an autosomal recessive disorder

42. A 56-year-old woman has a Chvostek's sign and Trousseau's sign on exam. She most likely has

    (A) hypercalcemia
    (B) hypokalemia
    (C) hypoglycemia
    (D) hypomagnesemia
    (E) hypothyroidism

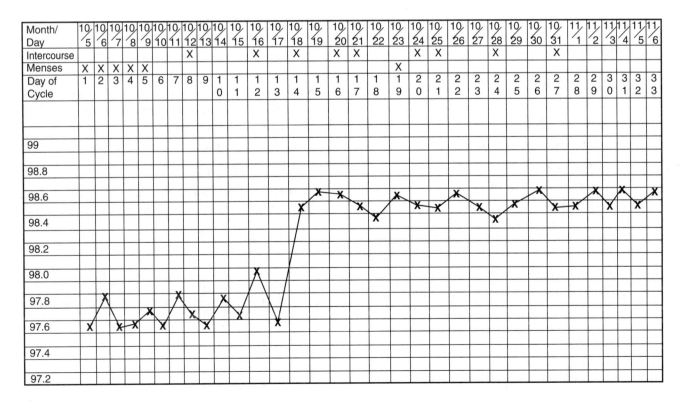

Figure 4.3

43. What is the etiologic agent of condyloma acuminata?

    (A) human papillomavirus
    (B) poxvirus
    (C) echovirus
    (D) herpes simplex virus
    (E) parvovirus

Questions 44 through 46

You are asked to provide a consultation on a 31-year-old male patient with a 2-year history of nausea, vomiting, and diarrhea that are partially relieved with over-the-counter H_2 antagonists. There is no history of weight loss and no family history. The patient has undergone previous esophagogastroduodenoscopy (EGD) that revealed no ulcerations. Physical examination is unrevealing. Hemoglobin, hematocrit, and red blood cell (RBC) indices are within normal limits.

44. Which of the following diagnostic tests should be performed next?

    (A) repeat EGD and biopsy for *H. pylori*
    (B) esophageal manometry and 24-hour esophageal pH probe
    (C) gastric analysis
    (D) bentiromide test
    (E) swallowing function study

45. Which of the following serum tests would be the most appropriate in this patient?

    (A) Schilling test
    (B) fasting serum gastrin
    (C) immunoglobulin test for *H. pylori*
    (D) amylase and lipase
    (E) colonoscopy

46. The patient underwent a surgical exploration, and a mass was resected from the submucosa of the duodenum. The patient was placed on a sufficient dose of proton pump inhibitor (PPI) to maintain his gastric acid secretory rate to less than 10 mEq/L/hr, and his symptoms resolved. You are asked to consult on this patient. Which of the following is the best management plan for this patient, assuming that the gastric acid hypersecretion is well controlled on medical therapy?

    (A) In the absence of diffuse metastatic disease by radiological imaging studies, surgical exploration should be performed.
    (B) Chemotherapy should be used as adjuvant therapy followed by surgical resection.
    (C) Radiation therapy combined with surgical resection should be performed if a tumor is localized by radiological imaging studies.
    (D) Metastatic tumor to the liver is best managed with radiation therapy.
    (E) no treatment at this point

47. Serum taken from a patient with Wegener's granulomatosis will often lead to a cytoplasmic staining pattern when indirect immunofluorescence probing for autoantibodies is performed on polymorphonuclear neutrophil cells. The specific target antigen that causes this immunofluorescent pattern is

    (A) myeloperoxidase
    (B) elastase
    (C) azurocidin
    (D) proteinase-3
    (E) amylase

48. Which of the following is a histopathologic feature that would favor the diagnosis of idiopathic pulmonary fibrosis or usual interstitial pneumonia?

    (A) fibroblast foci
    (B) uniform changes of fibrotic infiltrates
    (C) honeycombing with sparing of the subpleural regions
    (D) diffuse involvement of the lung
    (E) giant cells

49. What is the most common *direct* cause of maternal mortality in the United States?

    (A) hemorrhage
    (B) embolism
    (C) hypertension

(D) automobile accidents

(E) smoking

50. A 67-year-old hypertensive man presents with the acute onset, just 1 hour prior to his arrival in the ED, of left-sided homonymous hemianopsia, left body neglect, and loss of graphesthesia in the left hand. He has no motor weakness. Blood pressure is 160/100 and heart rate is 88 and regular. Routine lab work including platelet count and coagulation studies are normal. An urgent computed tomographic (CT) scan of the head is normal. Where is his anatomic lesion?

(A) right frontal lobe

(B) right parietal lobe

(C) right temporal lobe

(D) right occipital lobe

(E) right brain stem

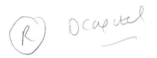

Answers and Explanations

1. **(C)** Complete removal of the thyroid gland results in hypothyroidism. The recurrent laryngeal nerve is in close proximity to the thyroid gland and may become damaged during this procedure. Tetany may occur as a manifestation of severe hypocalcemia, which may result from damage to the parathyroid glands located posterior to the thyroid. Hypercalcemia is not a complication of total thyroidectomy.

2. **(D)** The diagnosis is most consistent with CML. This, however, could be CLL, but generally the platelet count is low rather than high, which is more suggestive of a myeloproliferative disorder. This could easily be distinguished by a peripheral smear.

3. **(D)** Nonsteroidal anti-inflammatory drugs (NSAIDs) can produce a clinical picture suggestive of porphyria cutanea tarda with a normal porphyrin screen.

4. **(C)** Pseudomembranous colitis represents a full-blown manifestation of *C. difficile* colitis. It is characterized by sigmoidoscopic evidence of classic pseudomembranes, which appear as raised yellow or off-white plaques ranging up to 1 cm in diameter scattered over the colonic mucosa. Pseudomembranes are not associated with the other organisms listed.

5. **(D)** The most important step in the treatment of diarrhea induced by *C. difficile* is cessation of the inciting antibiotic. In general, the most commonly associated antibiotics are the cephalosporins, ampicillin, and clindamycin. Patients with mild symptoms are usually treated with vancomycin or metronidazole. Oral metronidazole (Flagyl) is administered at a dose of 500 mg TID. An alternative agent is oral vancomycin at a dose of 125 mg QID. It should be noted that both agents are equally effective and metronidazole is less expensive to adminster than vancomycin.

6. **(D)** Severe vitamin C deficiency results in scurvy. It occurs in severely malnourished individuals whose diet includes less than 10 mg/day of vitamin C. It is usually seen in association with drug or alcohol abuse, poverty, or in chronically ill and institutionalized patients. Collagen synthesis requires ascorbic acid as a cofactor for the formation of hydroxyproline and hydroxylysine, and is therefore essential for wound healing. Clinical syndromes are largely related to this impaired collagen synthesis and classically include ecchymoses, splinter hemorrhages, bleeding gums, and hyperkeratotic hair follicles with surrounding perifollicular hyperemia or hemorrhage. They may also have arthritis, edema, neuropathy, and vasomotor instability. Although vitamin K deficiency can manifest as a bleeding disorder, the peculiar perifollicular distribution and hyperkeratosis are nearly pathognomonic for vitamin C deficiency.

7. **(C)** This is consistent with the clinical picture of TTP. Generally, patients have varying neurological signs, fragmentation hemolytic anemia, fever, renal abnormalities, and thrombocytopenia. Most patients with this

disease are women (~70%). It is generally treated with steroids and plasmapheresis.

8. **(E)** The counterregulatory response to hypoglycemia involves a variety of mechanisms. Glucagon is released from the pancreas and increases hepatic glucose release by stimulating glycogenolysis and gluconeogenesis. ACTH and cortisol are stimulated by hypoglycemia. Cortisol increases lipolysis, protein catabolism, and gluconeogenesis. Both the sympathetic and parasympathetic nervous systems are activated by hypoglycemia. Catecholamines produce warning symptoms such as palpitations, shaking, and sweating that warn the patient of hypoglycemia. They also increase glycogenolysis and gluconeogenesis and increase plasma free fatty acids. Vagal stimulation induces a hunger sensation.

9. **(E)** While pregnancy "wheels" are often used in the calculation of an EDD, the use of Nägele's rule gives an accurate estimation of an EDD and can be done in your head. To apply Nägele's rule for the calculation of an EDD, count back 3 months from the first day of the LMP and add 7 days. Obviously, the patient could not deliver a baby prior to becoming pregnant, making A an incorrect choice.

10. **(B)** Figure 4.2 is a picture of a Lewy body. Lewy bodies were formerly believed to be pathogenic for Parkinson's disease. These pathologic findings are now known to be associated with "Lewy-body disease" in which a slowly progressive dementia is associated with prominent psychosis with worsening when treated with phenothiazines. Wilson's disease is a disorder of copper metabolism affecting the basal ganglia, cornea (Kayser-Fleischer ring), and liver with a decrease of serum ceruloplasmin. Huntington's chorea is an autosomal dominant condition characterized by choreiform movement, dementia, and depression.

11. **(C)** The ACL prevents anterior translation of the tibia on the femur. ACL tears are more common in noncontact sports. Stop-and-jump and plant-and-pivot mechanisms of injury are the most common. Early emphasis on hamstring strengthening will reduce instability symptoms. The quadriceps and gastrocnemius should be strengthened following knee injury to restore normal gait.

12. **(C)** The impulse is generated in the atrium at the sinus node, passes along specialized atrial conduction tissue, through the AV node and His bundle. At the point that the impulse reaches the ventricle, the QRS is inscribed. A prolonged PR interval can result in delay anywhere along the route. A narrow complex following a long PR suggests proximal (or AV node) delay. A wide QRS following a long PR interval suggests the possibility of distal conduction system disease.

13. **(D)** Autosomal dominant polycystic kidney disease is a systemic disease with varied renal pathology, including renal cysts, calculi, infection, hemorrhage, and eventual renal insufficiency. Associated gastrointestinal pathology includes hepatic and pancreatic cysts. These patients also have an increased incidence of cerebral artery aneurysms. The cysts eventually become isolated structures, and standard empiric antibiotics for pyelonephritis penetrate cysts poorly. Lipid-soluble antibiotics are required and include trimethoprim, tetracycline, doxycycline, norfloxacin, and chloramphenicol. Ampicillin, aminoglycosides, and nitrofurantoin are not lipid soluble and thus are poor choices. Cephalosporins are soluble in water.

14. **(D)** The combination of high insulin and low C peptide is consistent with insulin use. In insulinoma and sulfonylurea use, insulin and C peptide are both high. In adrenal insufficiency and growth hormone deficiency, insulin and C peptide are both low.

15. **(A)** In MEN 1, there is a combination of pituitary, parathyroid, and pancreatic tumors. In MEN 2A, there is a combination of pheochromocytoma, hyperparathyroidism, and medullary thyroid carcinoma. In MEN 2B, there is a combination of pheochro-

mocytoma, medullary thyroid carcinoma, mucosal neuromas, and marfanoid habitus. MEN 3 and 4 do not exist.

16. **(C)** Signet cells are seen in Krukenberg's tumors, an adenocarcinoma metastatic to the ovary. Granulosa cells are seen in normal ovarian follicles and granulosa cell tumors. Sertoli-Leydig cells are seen in the rare ovarian androblastoma. Squamous cells are commonly seen in mature cystic teratomas or dermoid cysts. Immature neural tissue is seen in the malignant immature teratoma.

17. **(A)** The most common primary source of metastatic disease to the ovary is the breast. Colon and endometrial cancers also may spread to the ovaries. However, signet cell–containing Krukenberg-type tumors almost all start in the stomach.

18. **(C)** Low back pain is the most common cause of work-related disability. Prolonged sitting at work, obesity, vibrational stress, gender, and psychosocial issues are also risk factors. Walking is of benefit to overall physical health and can improve low back problems.

19. **(C)** Clindamycin may cause pseudomembranous colitis. The syndrome, which may be fatal, is apparently due to the production of an endotoxin by clindamycin-resistant strains of *C. difficile*. If significant diarrhea occurs, clindamycin should be discontinued. Agents that inhibit peristalsis, such as opiates, should not be given because they prolong and worsen the condition. The most active drugs against *C. difficile* are vancomycin and metronidazole administered for 7 to 14 days. Since metronidazole is also an alternative to clindamycin for the treatment of serious anaerobic infections, it would be the appropriate choice for this patient. Cefoxitin and cholestyramine are less effective.

20. **(D)** hCG is produced by the placenta and is detectable at about 3 weeks' gestation. It peaks during the tenth week of gestation, af-

ter which it declines gradually. Before the sixth week, the ovarian corpus luteum maintains the pregnancy by secreting progesterone and estrogen. After the seventh week, the placenta produces adequate estrogen and progesterone secretion to maintain the pregnancy, and therefore an oophorectomy would not result in abortion after this time. Follicle-stimulating and luteinizing hormone levels are suppressed throughout the pregnancy. hPL, which contributes to changes in maternal glucose and fatty acid metabolism, appears in serum at about 4 weeks and continues to rise until delivery. Prolactin also continues to rise throughout the pregnancy, and levels peak at delivery.

21. **(C)** Cortisol is a steroid hormone, whereas glucagon is a polypeptide hormone. About 90% of cortisol circulates bound to serum proteins (cortisol-binding globulin and albumin). Glucagon does not circulate in a protein-bound state. Both hormones stimulate gluconeogenesis. Glucagon stimulates glycogenolysis, whereas cortisol inhibits it. Both hormones are stimulated by hypoglycemia.

22. **(E)** A young woman with splenomegaly and vague low back and hip pain has Gaucher's disease. Bony lesions are quite commonly caused by infiltration with Gaucher's cells, which are macrophages filled with glucocerebroside.

23. **(B)** This patient presents with systemic vasculitis with intestinal ischemia due to obliterative endarteritis and, by pathology, granuloma formation involving intestinal medium-sized vessels. It would be incorrect in the setting of an ileus to perform either a percutaneous liver biopsy or colonoscopy, although both may yield a diagnosis of polyarteritis nodosa associated with mixed cryoglobulinemia involving either the liver or large intestine, respectively. Obtaining serum cryoglobulin levels or a cryocrit, although helpful in the diagnosis, would not be useful in diagnosing intestinal ischemia.

24. **(C)** MVP is a relatively frequently seen cause of cardiac valve abnormality with a 3% to 5% incidence. The leaflet(s), which may be congenitally redundant, prolapse into the left atrium during systole when the valve should be closed. The redundant leaflets and prolapse of the valve can cause tension on the chord and result in their rupture. This can lead to acute severe MVP. Patents with MVP can be asymptomatic to highly symptomatic and may develop ventricular arrhythmias. Patients with MVP and resultant mitral regurgitation should receive antibiotic prophylaxis.

25. **(B)** A Lisch nodule is a lesion of the iris that is one of the stigmata of neurofibromatosis. The nodule most likely represents a benign melanocytic hamartoma of neural crest origin. It may be located superficially or deep within the stroma of the iris.

26. **(C)** Patients with ulcerative colitis (UC) are not at increased risk for developing primary biliary cirrhosis. Patients with UC are at increased risk for developing sclerosing cholangitis and gallstones. The best diagnostic test for diagnosing sclerosing cholangitis is by ERCP, whereas a functional diagnostic exam such as with HIDA has a high sensitivity for diagnosing acute cholecystitis.

27. **(A)** Bethanecol is a stimulator of cholinergic receptors expressed on the smooth muscles of the gastrointestinal (GI) tract. Morphine sulfate is an opioid agonist and can result in slower motility. H_2-receptor antagonists block H_2 receptors expressed on the parietal cell and thereby result in a reduction of gastric acid secretion but have no effects on motility. Dopamine receptors are expressed in the central nervous system (CNS) and to a lesser extent in the periphery. Dopamine receptor antagonists would result in a reduction in bowel motility.

28. **(B)** A lumbar burst fracture is generally a stable spine injury and includes widening of the pedicles, retropulsion of the posterior vertebral body, vertebral body compression and neurologic impairment. The need for decompression and fusion depends on the extent of posterior body retropulsion and the degree of neurologic deficit. A patient with one-third canal compromise and a normal neurologic exam can usually be treated without surgery. A patient with canal compromise of 50% and an increasing lower extremity motor deficit is a surgical emergency.

29. **(E)** Axial loading directs forces radially in an outward direction, resulting in separation of the pedicles and retropulsion of the posterior body of the vertebrae.

30. **(A)** The sartorius origin is on the anterior superior iliac spine and its insertion is on the medial aspect of the proximal tibia.

31. **(A)** Asthma is far more common in children and young adults. The bone loss that can lead to osteoporosis accelerates at menopause. The other conditions are not related to menopause.

32. **(D)** Choices A, B, and C represent primary pleural effusions in which drainage of the effusion would allow for reexpansion of the lung. In these situations, the atelectasis of the lung would be secondary to compression from the effusion. However, if the atelectasis were the initial event from an obstructing endobronchial lesion, as can occur with bronchogenic carcinomas, then a passive secondary effusion may occur. Drainage of the effusion in this situation may not lead to reexpansion of the lung since the endobronchial obstruction remains.

33. **(B)** The 10-year history of a nongrowing lesion is most suggestive of a benign process. The fluctuance of the mass is consistent with papillary cystadenoma or a Warthin's tumor. This accounts for 10% of benign salivary tumors.

34. **(A)** Lead toxicity produces a predominantly motor neuronopathy, while acrylamide is associated with distal axonal neuropathy. The chemotherapeutic agents cis-platinum and

taxotere are associated with predominantly sensory neuropathies. Cis-platinum affects large sensory fibers (vibration and proprioception), while taxotere causes a painful small-fiber neuropathy.

35. **(B)**   This is the typical pathology of a patient with dermatomyositis. The typical violaceous rash may appear later in the clinical course. Vasculitis should display inflammatory cells within the wall of the vessel, and polymyositis does not display a perifascicular pattern of atrophy. Regenerating and degenerating muscle cells are a hallmark of inflammatory myopathy. Rimmed vacuoles are commonly seen in patients with inclusion body myositis.

36. **(B)**   The effects on disease progression have been modest but statistically significant. Many patients and families have noted improved cognitive abilities as well.

37. **(B)**   Indications for PCI or CABG include suitable multivessel disease, but CABG alone is appropriate for unprotected left main artery disease. Repeat CABG is an option in patients with prior bypass operations.

38. **(A)**   Alpha$_1$-antitrypsin deficiency is a hereditary cause of emphysema, particularly in the setting of smoking. The MM phenotype is most common and normal. The abnormal ZZ phenotype is the most common cause of clinically significant alpha$_1$-antitrypsin deficiency. The abnormal alpha$_1$-antitrypsin made in the liver polymerize and accumulates in the hepatocytes, with decreased secretion of functional alpha$_1$-antitrypsin into circulation. The accumulation eventually is injurious to the liver and can lead to cirrhosis. With the null phenotype, there can be severe emphysema because there is no protective antiproteolytic effects of alpha$_1$-antitrypsin at all; however, no liver disease occurs since there is no accumulation of an abnormal alpha$_1$-antitrypsin variant.

39. **(C)**   When the basal body temperature remains elevated for more than 14 days after presumed ovulation (around the time of initial rise in temperature), especially in a patient actively trying to conceive, pregnancy is likely. No consistent midcycle temperature rise is seen with anovulation. FUO is associated with temperature above 38°C (100.4°F). Luteal-phase defect is associated with a shortened luteal phase, which would be reflected by a temperature rise after ovulation of less than 14 days' duration.

40. **(C)**   In general, the most common malignant tumor of the oropharynx is squamous cell rather than adenocarcinoma. They tend to occur in smokers, and alcohol has been found to be synergistic. They often metastasize to local lymph nodes, making treatment difficult. Multifocal or advanced-stage tumors have a poor prognosis.

41. **(A)**   Arrhythmias have been associated with MVP. Sudden death is uncommon without mitral regurgitation (MR) but up to 1.9% present with MR. The abnormal connective tissue may be inherited as an autosomal dominant gene with variable penetrance. The auscultatory findings typically include an apical midsystolic nonejection click and late systolic murmur of MR.

42. **(D)**   Hypomagnesemia leads to hypocalcemia, which causes both signs on exam. Chvostek's is the twitching of the circumoral muscles in response to tapping the facial nerve. Trousseau's is the carpal spasm elicited by inflation of a blood pressure cuff to 20 mmHg above the patient's systolic pressure.

43. **(A)**   Human papillomavirus is the etiologic agent for genital warts (condyloma acuminata).

44–46. **(44-C, 45-B, 46-A)**   The patient presents with Zollinger-Ellison syndrome (ZES). The best single diagnostic study in gastric acid hypersecretion is gastric analysis. EGD is frequently unrevealing in patients with Zollinger-Ellison syndrome, and evaluation for *H. pylori* is usually negative; therefore, repeat EGD and biopsy for *H. pylori* is incorrect. Esophageal manometry and 24-hour pH analysis are abnormal in only a small percentage of patients with ZES. The bentiromide test is not a useful test in ZES. The most sensitive serum assay is the fasting serum gastrin. There is no evidence that the patient presented has vitamin malabsorption; therefore, Schilling test is incorrect. There are no signs or symptoms to suggest that the patient is infected with *H. pylori*; therefore, an immunoglobulin study would not be indicated. Similarly, there is no evidence that the patient has acute pancreatitis; therefore, measurement of serum amylase or lipase would not be indicated in this patient.

In approximately 60% of patients with ZES, the dose of PPI can be safely reduced. In sporadic ZES, the tumor is localized to either the pancreas or duodenum in 80% of patients. Serum gastrin values are elevated in > 95% of patients with ZES. Patients with sporadic ZES not undergoing curative resection develop metastatic disease and a reduced survival. The least likely study to localize gastrinoma is an ERCP because most gastrinomas occur in either the duodenum or pancreas.

A bone scan is indicated in evaluating bone metastases. Endoscopic ultrasound is sensitive for detecting duodenal and pancreatic tumors. SRS and MRI are sensitive for detecting hepatic metastases. Surgical exploration should be performed in all patients with nonmetastatic sporadic ZES. Neither chemotherapy nor radiation therapy have been shown to be useful in the therapy of ZES.

47. **(D)** Several target antigens have been recognized to cause an ANCA (anti-neutrophil cytoplasmic autoantibody) pattern when performed by indirect immunofluorescence. When antigen-specific testing is performed by enzyme-linked immunosorbent assay (ELISA) methods, the characteristic cytoplasmic ANCA (c-ANCA) pattern can be attributed to proteinase-3 in Wegner's granulomatosis. Microscopic polyangiitis (MPA), like Wegener's granulomatosis is another systemic vasculitis that can manifest with a pulmonary–renal syndrome and also exhibits an ANCA pattern, but more specifically, the perinuclear-ANCA (p-ANCA) pattern. This pattern is less specific, but in patients with MPA, the most common target antigen is myeloperoxidase.

48. **(A)** Idiopathic pulmonary fibrosis is a cause of a progressive fibrotic lung disease with a dismal prognosis. No clear etiology or treatment is currently available. The histologic correlate to this diagnosis is usual interstitial pneumonia (UIP). Characteristic features of UIP include presence of fibroblast foci, honeycombing representing terminal lung disease, heterogeneous distribution of disease (normal lung next to diseased lung), predilection for the subpleura and lower lung zones, and temporal heterogeneity (interstitial changes seemingly at different stages of fibrosis). This diagnosis can occasionally be made based on a classic clinical, physiologic (pulmonary function tests), and radiographic (high-resolution CT) presentation.

49. **(B)** Motor vehicle accidents are not a direct cause of maternal mortality. If a woman is killed in a car accident while she is pregnant, this is considered to be a nonmaternal death. While hypertension and hemorrhage are more common complications of pregnancy in general, they are less often associated with maternal death.

50. **(B)** While a homonymous hemianopsia may be seen with lesions in the right occipital lobe, the associated neglect and agraphesthesia place this lesion in the parietal lobe. Astereognosis and sensory extinction, along with agraphesthesia, are the "cortical" sensory signs. When administered within the first 3 hours after an acute stroke, tissue plasminogen activator has been shown to reduce the eventual disability. There have been no studies proving any acute benefit to stroke outcome for the other therapies listed.

Practice Test 5
Questions

1. Proton pump inhibitors (PPIs) inhibit gastric acid secretion by which of the following mechanisms?

    (A) competitive antagonists of the gastrin receptor
    (B) competitive antagonists of the histamine 2 (H_2) receptor
    (C) direct inhibition of the H+,K+ ATPase
    (D) neutralization of gastric acidity
    (E) neutralization of the gastrin molecule

2. Figure 5.1 represents a thyroid cell. Which of the labeled sites is stimulated by thyroid-stimulating hormone (TSH)?

    (A) only A
    (B) only B
    (C) only D
    (D) only E
    (E) all sites listed

3. A 13-year-old boy notes leg pain and swelling. An x-ray is performed, and the affected limb reveals the classic sign of Codman's triangle. What is the most likely diagnosis?

    (A) chondrosarcoma
    (B) multiple myeloma

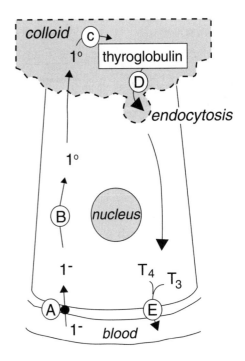

Figure 5.1

    (C) osteomyelitis
    (D) osteosarcoma
    (E) bone cyst

4. Injury to which of the following nerves results in "winging" of the scapula?

    (A) spinal accessory
    (B) long thoracic
    (C) axillary
    (D) musculocutaneous
    (E) suprascapular

5. A 65-year-old woman with breast cancer treated with surgical lumpectomy, radiation, and chemotherapy 3 years ago is seen in follow- up. She is found to have a hemoglobin of 8.2 g/dL but is completely asymptomatic. The most likely explanation is

(A) chemotherapy-induced marrow aplasia
(B) acute leukemia
(C) metastatic breast cancer
(D) iron deficiency
(E) indeterminate

6. What is the most common location of a venous leg ulceration?

(A) medial malleolus
(B) lateral malleolus
(C) knee
(D) heel
(E) base of great toe

7. The transient loss of motor amplitude (Figure 5.2) observed with low-rate repetitive stimulation of the ulnar nerve may be diagnostic of

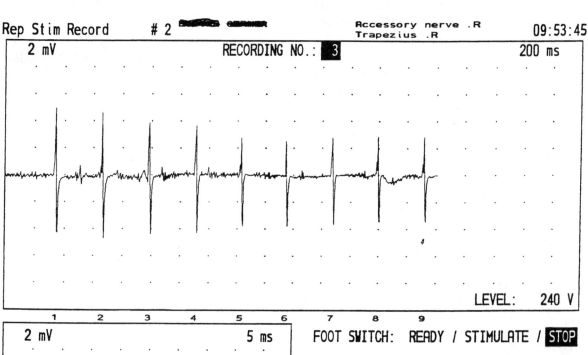

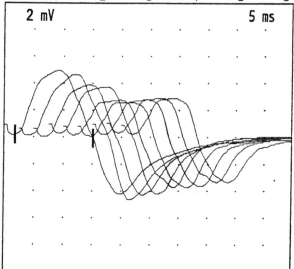

POT NO.	PEAK AMP mV	AMP. DECR %	AREA mVms	AREA DECR %	STIM. LEVEL
1	4.77	0	40.60	0	240V
2	4.52	5	37.40	8	240V
3	3.84	19	30.80	24	240V
4	3.46	27	31.80	22	240V
5	2.59	46	24.10	41	240V
6	2.44	49	22.90	44	240V
7	2.57	46	24.40	40	240V
8	2.57	46	25.40	37	240V
9	2.65	44	25.30	38	240V

Figure 5.2

(A) Lambert-Eaton syndrome

(B) myasthenia gravis

(C) Guillain-Barré syndrome

(D) botulism

(E) tetanus

8. A patient with pseudohypoparathyroidism will most likely have which of the following physical features?

(A) tall stature

(B) polydactyly

(C) webbed neck

(D) exophthalmos

(E) short fourth and fifth metacarpals

9. A patient has a bronchoscopy performed due to unexplained dyspnea and cough. On entering the trachea, the mucosa is inflamed, and there is collapse of a segment of the anterior wall with coughing. What is the likely diagnosis?

(A) dynamic airway collapse from severe asthma

(B) chronic bronchitis

(C) tracheomalacia

(D) herpes tracheitis

(E) asthma

10. A patient is seen in the clinic. On physical exam, the following findings were noted: The left ventricular impulse was nondisplaced. S1 and S2 were normal. A grade II/VI systolic murmur started after a short pause following S1 and ending before S2. The murmur was loudest in the fourth left intercostal space. These findings are consistent with

(A) mitral regurgitation

(B) tricuspid regurgitation

(C) mitral valve prolapse (MVP)

(D) innocent murmur

(E) aortic stenosis

11. Which of the following hormonal conditions is present during the midluteal (secretory) phase of the menstrual cycle?

(A) Luteinizing hormone (LH) and follicle-stimulating hormone (FSH) levels are peaking.

(B) Progesterone levels are at their lowest point.

(C) Viscosity of cervical mucus is low.

(D) The corpus luteum has been completely replaced by fibrous tissue.

(E) Low FSH and LH

12. A 58-year-old man presents with a white, scaly rash involving the palm of one hand and the soles of his feet. It is associated with moderate pruritus. What is the most likely diagnosis?

(A) tinea pedis/manus

(B) psoriasis

(C) ichthyosis

(D) atopic dermatitis

(E) allergic dermatitis

13. A positron emission tomographic (PET) study is ordered on a patient with a 1.5-cm lung nodule and mildly enlarged mediastinal lymph nodes to assess for malignant potential. Which of the following will likely lead to a false-negative PET scan?

(A) The lesion is due to small cell carcinoma.

(B) Patient is diabetic with a glucose level of 210 mg/dL.

(C) The nodule and adenopathy are due to active histoplasmosis.

(D) The nodule is a carcinoid tumor.

(E) The patient is a heavy smoker.

14. A 60-year-old patient on chronic hemodialysis continues to bleed after a radical prostatectomy. Laboratory studies reveal a normal platelet count, and activated partial thromboplastin time (aPTT) and prothrombin time (PT) were normal. This is due to

(A) thrombocytopenia

(B) inadequate levels of vitamin K

(C) hypofibrinogenemia

(D) thromboplastin deficiency

(E) a qualitative platelet defect

15. Hypergastrinemia (i.e., elevation in serum gastrin levels > 100 pg/mL) would be expected to occur in which of the following conditions?

    (A) Zollinger-Ellison syndrome
    (B) acute renal failure
    (C) short-term use of PPIs
    (D) Barrett's esophagus
    (E) manic depression

16. A 20-year-old patient has pseudohypoparathyroidism. When she was initially diagnosed at age 12, she had which of the following combinations of laboratory tests?

	Serum Calcium	Serum Phosphate	Serum Parathyroid Hormone
(A)	High	Low	High
(B)	Low	High	High
(C)	Low	Low	High
(D)	High	High	High
(E)	Low	Low	Low

17. A 65-year-old man with a 60-pack-year history of smoking and an extensive alcohol history including 1 case of beer/day is noted to have increased lower extremity edema, with 3–4+ pitting for 2 months. The evaluation of this patient should include

    (A) chest x-ray and serum albumin
    (B) renal biopsy
    (C) barium enema
    (D) examination of all extremity joints
    (E) all body parts from the neck down

18. A 65-year-old retired physician received a purified protein derivative (PPD) as part of the application process for a volunteer job. The induration of the PPD is 17 mm in 48 hours, with his last PPD 5 years ago being negative. He denies any symptoms or definite exposures to tuberculosis and is initiated on isoniazid therapy. Eight months into therapy, he returns with complaints of persistent diarrhea. He has also had nausea and emesis. His wife reports that the patient has been recently confused. Examination reveals an anxious man who is mildly disoriented and a prominent erythematous rash in a photodistribution. There is no evidence of peripheral neuropathy. What is the likely cause of this patient's symptoms?

    (A) vitamin A deficiency
    (B) vitamin A toxicity
    (C) vitamin B_{12} deficiency
    (D) vitamin C deficiency
    (E) niacin deficiency

19. A 40-year-old man presents to your practice complaining of tenderness in the anal canal for 1 week. The patient denied symptomatic improvement following sitz bath and suppositories. On examination the patient was afebrile, and a rectal examination revealed exquisite tenderness of the anal canal. Anoscopy revealed no blood or purulent drainage. Which of the following conditions would be unexpected?

    (A) perianal abscess
    (B) Crohn's disease
    (C) internal hemorrhoids
    (D) pilonidal cyst
    (E) anal fistula

20. A 35-year-old woman presents with headaches and galactorrhea and is found to have a 2-cm mass in her pituitary gland. Blood work reveals markedly elevated prolactin levels. Which of the following medications will most likely improve her symptoms?

    (A) metoclopramide
    (B) reserpine
    (C) bromocriptine
    (D) methyldopa
    (E) risperidol

21. A study evaluating a new drug "X" is released. It has been purported to be beneficial in the prevention of acute renal failure following intravenous contrast administration in patients with mild renal insufficiency. However, it has several adverse reactions, some of which can be severe. The study involved 200 patients randomized to standard care versus standard care plus administration of this new drug. The results are demonstrated in the following table. What is the "number needed to treat" and the "number needed to harm"?

    (A) 10 and 5
    (B) 20 and 5
    (C) 10 and 20
    (D) 20 and 20
    (E) 40 and 40

22. A 24-year-old woman presents to your office and is found to have dermatitis, nail atrophy, a pancreatic mass, and elevated glucose on fingerstick. You suspect which of the following?

    (A) glucagonoma
    (B) hepatoma
    (C) lipoma
    (D) glucola
    (E) pancreatitis

23. Which of the following patients would have the highest risk for the development of adenocarcinoma of the esophagus?

    (A) a 40-year-old woman with a history of excessive coffee drinking and a 20-pack-year history of cigarette smoking
    (B) a 70-year-old African-American man with a history of excessive exposure to alcohol and cigarettes
    (C) a 50-year-old white man with no history of drinking alcohol
    (D) a 62-year-old woman with a 40-year history of drinking alcohol
    (E) a 23-year-old factory worker with dust exposure

24. A 58-year-old woman with a long history of severe psoriasis necessitating systemic therapy is diagnosed with pulmonary fibrosis. Which of the following drugs is the most likely cause?

    (A) cyclosporine
    (B) methotrexate
    (C) acitretin
    (D) etanercept
    (E) prednisolone

25. Proton pump inhibitors (PPIs) would inhibit which of the following?

    (A) histamine
    (B) somatostatin
    (C) H+,K+ ATPase
    (D) pepsinogen
    (E) serotonin

26. A 22-year-old sexually active man presents with a several-week history of right inguinal groin pain and severe anal pain. On examination there are shallow ulcerations noted in the anal canal and exquisite tenderness noted in the perianal area. Bilateral, enlarged inguinal lymph nodes are present. Which of the following is the most likely diagnosis?

    (A) perianal abscess
    (B) perianal fissure
    (C) herpes simplex infection
    (D) *Cryptosporidium* infection
    (E) staph dermatitis

27. A 58-year-old woman is on multiple medications for management of her diabetes. One day after skipping her lunch, she developed light-headedness and found her blood glucose to be 40 mg/dL. Which of the following medications is most likely to cause hypoglycemia?

    (A) metformin
    (B) pioglitazone
    (C) acarbose
    (D) glipizide
    (E) digoxin

28. A 59-year-old woman presents to your office complaining of a 2-month history of early satiety and abdominal bloating. On pelvic exam you detect a 6-cm right adnexal mass and mild abdominal distention with an air–fluid wave on abdominal exam. Subsequent pelvic ultrasound shows a complex right adnexal mass with a normal left adnexa and uterus, as well as a moderate amount of ascites and neoplasias, including choriocarcinoma. Alpha-fetoprotein (AFP) may be elevated with the less common endodermal sinus tumors. Endodermal sinus tumors are germ cell tumors and usually are diagnosed in younger women. At the time of surgery, grossly apparent subcentimeter studding over the peritoneum, including the peritoneal surface of the liver, is observed along with tumor excrescenses over the surface of the enlarged, multicystic right ovary. Ascites is found on opening the abdomen and is sent for cytologic evaluation. The omentum is grossly studded with small (< 2 cm) tumor implants. The liver appears otherwise normal at surgery as well as on preoperative abdominal imaging. A preoperative chest x-ray was normal. The uterus and pelvic lymph nodes as well as the left ovary, are grossly and microscopically normal. Pathology on the right ovarian mass as well as peritoneal and omental implants are consistent with malignancy. Psammoma bodies are also noted in the ovarian tumor on microscopic examination. Cytologic examination of the ascitic fluid is positive for malignant cells. What is the correct diagnosis for this patient?

(A) Krukenberg's tumor
(B) granulosa cell tumor
(C) serous cystadenoma
(D) endodermal sinus tumor
(E) papillary serous cystadenocarcinoma

29. You are evaluating a 45-year-old man who was hospitalized for management of a variceal hemorrhage, and the patient's condition has stabilized with endoscopic therapy and blood transfusion. Preceding the hospitalization, the patient reports a history of malaise, fatigue, weight gain, and an increase in abdominal girth. The physical examination confirms the presence of ascites. There was no prior history of excessive alcohol ingestion, and the patient had tested negative for hepatitis C by history.

Laboratory Studies

Hemoglobin	11 g/dL
Platelet count	62,000/mm^3
Prothrombin time	16 seconds (control 12)
Serum ferritin	200 ng/mL

What would be the most appropriate course of action?

(A) Refer the patient for a liver transplantation consultation.
(B) Start alpha-interferon therapy.
(C) Perform a liver biopsy followed by interferon therapy.
(D) Send a ceruloplasmin level.
(E) Send home and reevaluate in 6 weeks.

30. In a woman with amenorrhea and high LH and FSH levels, what is the most likely diagnosis?

(A) pituitary insufficiency
(B) pregnancy
(C) primary ovarian failure
(D) abnormal gonadotropin-releasing hormone (GnRH) secretion
(E) ovarian cysts

31. A 30-year-old man with renal insufficiency presents with a urethral discharge and frequency of urination. Which antimicrobial agent can be used at the usual dosage in an azotemic patient?

(A) nitrofurantoin
(B) sulfisoxazole
(C) doxycycline
(D) trimethoprim
(E) fluconazole

32. A patient is seen in the clinic. On physical exam, the following findings were noted: A harsh late-peaking holosystolic murmur is heard starting after a soft S1. No S2 is heard. A thrill is palpable on the precordium. An S4 is present. The carotid pulse is slowly rising and the amplitude is small. These findings are consistent with which of the following?

(A) mitral regurgitation
(B) tricuspid regurgitation
(C) mitral valve prolapse
(D) innocent murmur
(E) aortic stenosis

33. The newer class of arthritic medications known as COX-2 nonsteroidal anti-inflammatory agents (NSAIDs) act by which of the following mechanisms?

(A) stimulate cyclooxygenase-2 production and, therefore, prostaglandin synthesis
(B) stabilize monocyte lysosomal membranes, preventing release of destructive cytokines
(C) prevent the multiplication of monocyte and neutrophil stem cells, which form part of the destructive pannus
(D) inhibit cyclooxygenase-2 and, therefore, prostaglandin synthesis
(E) inhibit histamine release

34. An elderly male who presents with a lower extremity ulcer and claudication would suggest what etiology for the ulcer?

(A) venous
(B) arterial
(C) neuropathic
(D) traumatic
(E) infectious

35. A 65-year-old woman with a history of rheumatoid arthritis presents with an upper GI bleed. The patient had been taking naproxen sodium at a dose of 500 mg tid for the past several years for her rheumatoid arthritis. An endoscopic examination was performed and showed a clean-based ulcer. The single best approach for the management of this patient is to

(A) continue the naproxen and start an H_2 receptor antagonist twice daily
(B) continue the naproxen and check a serum *Helicobacter pylori* antibody test
(C) admit the patient to the intensive care unit (ICU) and observe for signs of additional bleeding
(D) discontinue napoxen and start a PPI
(E) switch to ibuprofen 800 mg TID

36. Which of the following microscopic examinations is utilized to identify scabies?

(A) potassium hydroxide preparation
(B) Gram stain
(C) Tzanck preparation
(D) oil mount
(E) darkfield

37. A 49-year-old man is undergoing a routine annual examination. On review of systems, he reports excessive daytime sleepiness. His spouse notes that he has disruptive snoring and requires multiple naps throughout the day. She has also had to drive on distance trips as he has had extreme difficulty staying awake while driving. An overnight polysomnography reveals normal baseline saturations but marked desaturations occurring with numerous apneic and hypopneic events. The diagnosis of obstructive sleep apnea (OSA) is made. Which of the following would be an ineffective mode of treatment?

(A) nocturnal continuous positive airway pressure (CPAP) therapy
(B) restriction of body position during sleep
(C) nocturnal oxygen
(D) weight loss
(E) surgery

38. A 40-year-old man presents with a history of an upper GI bleed. The patient denied having a history of prior ulcer disease, NSAID use, and alcohol or tobacco use. The past medical history is unremarkable. The patient denies taking medications. There is no family history of ulcer disease. An endoscopy revealed a large jejunal ulcer with a visible vessel and duodenal and esophageal erosions. The following are pertinent laboratory and radiological studies:

Serum creatinine	1.2 mg/dL	Serum bilirubin	1.2 mg/dL
Hemoglobin	9.4 g/dL	Platelets	144,000/mm³
Leukocyte count	11,000/mm³		
Chest radiography	Normal		

The most likely diagnosis for this patient is

(A) *H. pylori* infection
(B) atrophic gastritis
(C) gastrinoma
(D) cytomegalovirus (CMV) infection
(E) potassium chloride ingestion

39. Following the onset of chest pain in acute myocardial infarction (MI), lactate dehydrogenase (LDH), troponin, and creatine kinase (CK) can be released from myocardial cells that suffer irreversible damage. On the graph

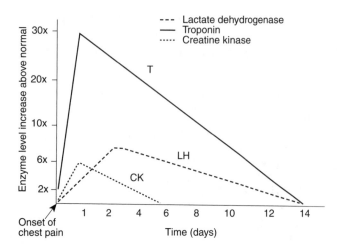

below, the correct time-line sequence for enzyme release following MI is:

(A) A = LDH, B = troponin, C = CK
(B) A = CK, B = LDH, C = troponin
(C) A = troponin, B = CK, C = LDH
(D) A = troponin, B = LDH, C = CK
(E) A = CK, B = LDH, C = troponin

40. A 64-year-old man is evaluated because a routine physical examination was performed, which included a stool examination for occult blood (hemoccult card test). The test result was positive for occult blood. A colonoscopy was then performed, and a pedunculated polyp was found in the descending colon, which revealed a poorly differentiated carcinoma invading the stalk. Which of the following would you recommend?

(A) repeat colonoscopy at 3 years
(B) repeat colonoscopy at 3 months
(C) referral to a surgeon for a partial colectomy
(D) referral to an oncologist for chemotherapy
(E) sigmoidoscopy in 3 months and colonoscopy in 1 year

41. A 45-year-old woman recently returned from a vacation in Mexico. After returning to the United States the patient noted crampy abdominal discomfort and an increase in the frequency of bowel movements. Later, she reports to you fever, malaise, watery diarrhea, and abdominal cramps. Examination shows no fever and is otherwise unremarkable except for orthostatic hypotension. Examination of the stools for ova and parasites and for occult blood is negative. Which of the following is the most likely diagnosis?

(A) *Vibrio cholera*
(B) enterotoxigenic *Escherichia coli*
(C) *Clostridium difficile*
(D) rotavirus
(E) *Listeria*

42. In the United States, currently available Food and Drug Administration (FDA)-approved emergency contraceptive pills can contain

    (A) misoprostol
    (B) mifepristone
    (C) diethylstilbestrol
    (D) prostaglandin E$_2$
    (E) levonorgestrel

43. Maternal administration of anti-D antibodies in the immediate postpartum period is used to prevent future pregnancy complications in

    (A) a mom with no antibody to rubella
    (B) a mom with an O negative blood type who gave birth to a baby with an A negative blood type
    (C) a mom with an O positive blood type who gave birth to a B positive baby
    (D) a mom with a B negative blood type who gave birth to an O positive baby
    (E) a mom who is not immune to chickenpox

44. The biceps femoris muscle originates from the

    (A) anterior superior iliac spine
    (B) anterior inferior iliac spine
    (C) supra-acetabular area of the ilium and the anterior inferior iliac spine
    (D) lateral iliac wing and posterior superior iliac spine
    (E) anterior aspect of the proximal femur

45. A patient has a friend who had a baby with spina bifida. She has heard that there is "something" she can take to decrease the chance of her baby's being affected by this problem. Which advice would you give the patient?

    (A) She is mistaken; there is no known way to prevent most birth defects.
    (B) Since she is 18 years old, it is very unlikely that she will have a baby with spina bifida.

    (C) It is too late for her to do anything to prevent this type of abnormality since the neural tube is closed in the first trimester of pregnancy.
    (D) Starting folic acid supplementation will lower her chance of having a baby with spina bifida.
    (E) Take B complex daily.

46. A 56-year-old man is diagnosed with squamous cell carcinoma of the lung. He is also hypercalcemic. After resection of the lung cancer, the calcium returns to normal. Which of the following was the cause of this patient's hypercalcemia?

    (A) PTH
    (B) 1,25-dihydroxyvitamin D
    (C) bone metastases
    (D) PTH-related protein
    (E) multivitamin abuse

47. A 32-year-old woman has high serum calcium and high PTH. She also has a history of prolactinoma and insulinoma. You resect her parathyroids. On reviewing the pathology slides of her parathyroid glands, which of the following findings would you see?

    (A) single adenoma
    (B) double adenomas
    (C) four-gland hyperplasia
    (D) carcinoma
    (E) excess beta cells

48. A pregnant patient confides to you that she had several beers at a party about 4 weeks ago. She also has an occasional beer (less than 1/week) for the past several weeks. You advise her

    (A) that her baby will most likely have mental retardation and hyperactivity

    (B) that there is no safe level of alcohol use established in pregnancy but it is only with heavy maternal alcohol use in the first trimester that any abnormalities in babies has been noted

    (C) that most women whose babies are born with fetal alcohol syndrome drink heavily throughout pregnancy

    (D) that alcohol use is safe in pregnancy as long as it is used in moderation and not drunk prior to driving

    (E) to increase the beer drinking frequency to avoid fetal alcohol withdrawal syndrome

49. Regarding myocarditis, which of the following statements is correct?

    (A) Myocarditis is a chronic disease manifested by a systemic inflammatory reaction.

    (B) The most common mechanism of injury is immunologic related to toxic exposures.

    (C) Symptoms are generally acute and severe.

    (D) The most common cause of myocarditis in the United States is viral.

    (E) Pain with myocarditis is positional.

50. Regarding neural regulation of the cardiac system, which of the following statements is correct?

    (A) With positional changes, there is compensatory vasodilation in the venous system.

    (B) Autonomic reflexes are activated through activation of baroreceptors in the aortic arch and carotid bodies.

    (C) Parasympathetic activation results in enhanced myocardial ontractility.

    (D) Drugs used to enhance the autonomic reflex mechanism and treat orthostasis include ganglionic blocking drugs.

    (E) Enhanced vasomotor tone is not due to sympathetic activation.

Answers and Explanations

1. **(C)** PPIs are substituted benzimidazoles that inhibit acid secretion by covalenly binding to the H+,K+-ATPase to block the movement of protons. These agents therefore do not competitively block either the gastrin receptor or the histamine 2 (H$_2$) receptor. Agents that directly neutralize of buffer gastric acidity would include antacids.

2. **(E)** TSH stimulates uptake of iodide by the thyroid cell, oxidation of iodide, and iodination of thyroglobulin. It also stimulates thyroglobulin resorption from colloid, secretion of thyroid hormones, and thyroid cell growth.

3. **(D)** When an osteogenic sarcoma penetrates the bony cortex, the periosteum becomes elevated, producing an angle with the underlying remaining cortical bone known as Codman's triangle. Thus, this finding is consistent with osteosarcoma.

4. **(B)** The serratus anterior muscle is innervated by the long thoracic nerve. Denervation of this muscle produces scapular winging when forward pushing movements are attempted. One common cause of long thoracic nerve dysfunction is a viral infection. This infection usually resolves spontaneously in 6 to 12 months.

5. **(E)** This patient could have all of the listed causes for her low hemoglobin, but the diagnosis cannot be made without further information such as a peripheral smear, further lab data, and a reticulocyte count. Older individuals may have nutritional deficiencies from inadequate diet and gastrointestinal (GI) blood loss from perhaps a secondary colon cancer. Metastatic tumors can produce a marrow replacement type of anemia. Chemotherapy-induced marrow failure can be prolonged in some cases. Secondary leukemias can occur from anthracycline-based chemotherapy. However, there is inadequate information to draw any conclusions.

6. **(A)** Venous leg ulcerations are characteristically located over the medial malleolus.

7. **(B)** In myasthenia gravis, due to the inactivation of postsynaptic neuromuscular junction acetylcholine receptors and depletion of the stores of presynaptic acetylcholine, there is an exhaustion of acetylcholine at low rates of stimulation. Botulinum toxin binds to the presynaptic membrane, preventing release of acetylcholine, while the Lambert-Eaton syndrome is an autoimmune disease in which an autoantibody inactivates the presynaptic calcium channels. Both of these latter conditions are characterized by a reduced amplitude of the resting compound motor action potential with an incremental response to high rates of repetitive stimulation.

8. **(E)** Patients with pseudohypoparathyroidism may have Albright's osteodystrophy: short stature, short fourth and fifth metacarpals, and a round face.

9. **(C)** The anatomy of the trachea is important to know in recognizing the abnormality during this patient's bronchoscopy. The cartilaginous skeleton of the trachea is typically "U"

shaped with the membranous (or the noncartilaginous) portion situated posteriorly. The cartilage provides rigidity to the airway and prevents collapse during respiration. With dynamic airway collapse rapid air flows such as with coughing, may elicit apparent "collapse" of the membranous portion of the trachea, but the anterior aspect of the trachea with the cartilaginous support should not. Therefore, the bronchoscopic finding suggests tracheomalacia, which can be related to several conditions, including relapsing polychondritis.

10. **(C)** Innocent murmurs are generally midsystolic and heard at the fourth left intercostal space. They can be from grade I to grade II/VI. There are no associated clicks, ejection sounds, or other murmurs.

11. **(E)** During the midluteal phase of the menstrual cycle, progesterone levels are at their highest. LH and FSH levels peaked at ovulation and are now low. The viscosity of cervical mucus is high. The corpus luteum is still present but will gradually be replaced by fibrous tissue and become nonfunctional by the end of the menstrual cycle.

12. **(A)** Acral tinea infections have a characteristic predilection for involvement of both feet and only one hand.

13. **(B)** The PET scan utilizes radioactive glucose to measure where glucose metabolism might be high. Since malignanices are metabolically active, they will typically show increased uptake by PET imaging. However, infections can also show abnormal uptake and will lead to a false positive. Because of the dependence of the PET scan on glucose utilization, a patient with an elevated glucose may have a false-negative study, making B the best answer. Slow-growing tumors, such as typical carcinoids or bronchioloalveolar cell carcinomas, also have the potential for false-negative PET studies.

14. **(E)** In patients with chronic renal failure, blood clothing is abnormal because of platelet dysfunction resulting from a defi-ciency of von Willebrand factor multimers and the presence of small molecules that impair platelet function. Because of the qualitative platelet defect, the most sensitive test to predict the occurrence of bleeding is the determination of a bleeding time.

15. **(A)** Elevation of serum gastriin (> 100 pg/mL) occurs commonly in patients diagnosed with Zollinger-Ellison syndrome due to the excessive release of gastrin from a gastrinoma tumor. Similarly, in patients with chronic renal failure or in those undergoing hemodialysis, gastrin levels are markedly elevated. This occurs because gastrin is renally excreted. Renal transplantation would be expected to normalize the serum gastrin levels. Patients chronically taking the potent acid inhibitors, PPIs, are likely to have mildly elevated gastrin levels. This occurs because there is often an increase in the enterochromaffin-like cell mass.

16. **(B)** In pseudohypoparathyroidism, there is resistance to parathyroid hormone (PTH), which leads to low calcium, high phosphate, and high PTH.

17. **(A)** In both a tobacco user and alcoholic, oral cavity and oropharynx cancers are quite common and need to be further investigated. In any patient with edema, serum albumin levels would be helpful. Liver failure could be a possibility, and liver function tests as well as assessment of the liver by CT should be done. A chest x-ray to assess the heart and presence of pulmonary edema should be done. In a chronic alcoholic, there is a predisposition to the development of hepatocellular carcinoma, and thus the CT would be helpful. A barium enema is not useful at this time.

18. **(E)** Isoniazid therapy can lead to an effective vitamin B_6 deficiency and manifest with peripheral neuropathy, ataxia, and paresthesias. However, this patient likely has developed pellagra (niacin deficiency), which manifests classically with a photodermatitis as with sunburns, diarrhea, and dementia. It is rare in industrialized countries except in alcoholics. In third-world countries, it may be associated

with local diets consisting primarily of corn, sorghum, or cereal. Three additional settings in which niacin deficiency is also possible include the prolonged use of isoniazid, malignant carcinoid, and Hartnup disease.

19. **(D)** This patient presents with a perianal abscess and anal fistula. The patient's condition may result from Crohn's disease. The differential diagnosis includes internal hemorrhoids. Pilonidal cyst is an unlikely diagnosis.

20. **(C)** Bromocriptine is an ergot alkaloid and a dopamine agonist. Dopamine and dopamine agonists inhibit synthesis and secretion of prolactin. They also inhibit proliferation of lactotrophs, which usually leads to tumor shrinkage. Metoclopramide, reserpine, methyldopa, and risperidol all antagonize dopamine and may increase prolactin levels.

21. **(A)** The number needed to treat (NNT) or the number needed to harm (NNH) is another way of evaluating the effect of treatments or interventions. It is often more intuitive and meaningful to the clinician than other measures such as the relative risk or odds ratios. The NNT is calculated by taking the inverse of the absolute risk reduction. Therefore, in our problem, the absolute risk reduction is 20/100 (standard care) minus 10/100 (drug X) which is 0.1. The NNT to treat is the reciprocal of this and is therefore 10. This means that 10 patients would need to be treated with drug X to prevent one acute renal failure. The NNH is similarly calculated. The absolute risk gain is 25/100 − 5/100 = 20/100 = 0.2. The NNH is the inverse of this and is therefore 5. This means that every five patients treated with drug X will have a serious adverse drug reaction as compared to standard therapy.

22. **(A)** Glucagonomas are associated with dermatitis, nail atrophy, pancreatic masses, and hyperglycemia. Gastric hypersecretion occurs with gastrinomas.

23. **(C)** Adenocarcinoma of the esophagus is increasing in prevalence, especially in white middle-aged men and in patients with a history of Barrett's esophagus. Smoking and alcohol are associated with the development of squamous cell cancers of the esophagus, especially in African-Americans.

24. **(B)** An adverse effect of methotrexate is a gradual pulmonary toxicity characterized as pulmonary fibrosis on chest x-ray.

25. **(C)** PPIs are a group of substituted benzimidazoles that, once activated by an acidic environment, are able to covalently bind to the H+,K+ ATPase and prevent the movement of H+ and K+ ions in the parietal cell.

26. **(C)** Perianal abscesses are generally accompanied by fever and radiating pain. On examination a tender mass may be present but no shallow ulcerations. Anal fissures are accompanied by exquisite pain, but ulcerations are absent. Herpes simplex infection may result in ulcerations and are accompanied by exquisite pain. *Cryptosporidium* causes colitis in immunocompromised and normal hosts but is not accompanied by ulcerations.

27. **(D)** Glipizide lowers blood glucose levels by stimulating the pancreatic beta cells to secrete insulin. One of the side effects of this medication is therefore hypoglycemia. Metformin and pioglitazone work by enhancing sensitivity to insulin in the liver and muscle cells. They do not raise insulin levels and therefore do not cause hypoglycemia on their own. Acarbose competitively inhibits the brush-border enzyme alpha-glucosidase to impede carbohydrate absorption. It does not cause hypoglycemia.

28. **(E)** Psammoma bodies are seen with the papillary serous ovarian neoplasms. Since the description is that of a malignant tumor, this would make papillary serous cystadenocarcinoma the correct diagnosis. Signet cells are the hallmark of the metastatic ovarian Krukenberg's tumor. Schiller-Duval bodies (tumor cells surrounding a single papillary projection with a central blood vessel) are seen with endodermal sinus tumors.

29. **(A)** This patient undoubtedly has cirrhosis, the etiology of which is unclear. Although the patient reports a negative test for hepatitis C, this test should be repeated and a confirmation test ordered. Whatever the cause of the cirrhosis, this otherwise young patient should be considered for a transplantation at some future time. Choice B is incorrect because the diagnosis of hepatitis C needs to be confirmed. Choice C would not confirm whether the patient is infected with hepatitis C and therefore is incorrect. Choice D, although helpful for establishing the diagnosis, would not provide therapy for the patient, and he would otherwise still require a transplant.

30. **(C)** In the absence of the ovarian production of estrogen and progesterone, as in primary ovarian failure, there is no feedback inhibition of pituitary gonadotropin secretion, and therefore LH and FSH levels are elevated. In amenorrhea caused by pituitary insufficiency, LH and FSH levels are diminished. In pregnancy, estrogen and progesterone both inhibit the release of LH and FSH. If hypothalamic GnRH is not secreted normally, LH and FSH cannot be secreted adequately from the pituitary gland.

31. **(C)** All the antibiotics listed—including most tetracyclines, except doxycycline—are excreted primarily in the urine, and blood levels increase in the presence of renal insufficiency.

32. **(E)** In severe aortic stenosis a harsh, late-peaking murmur is heard, which can be holosystolic. The second heart sound may be inaudible. A click can be heard if the valve remains mobile enough, but this finding is often not heard in severe aortic stenosis. An S4 is generally present preceding a soft S1. Pulsus parvus, a slow-rising pulse, is common. The amplitude of the pulse is diminished.

33. **(D)** COX-2 inhibitors have the advantage of a lower incidence of GI problems than the older NSAIDs. The COX-2 inhibitor celecoxib (Celebrex), unfortunately, is antigenically close enough to sulfa-based antibiotics to produce reactions in patients with allergy to sulfa drugs.

34. **(B)** The presence of claudication is characteristic of arterial insufficiency.

35. **(D)** The patient has endoscopic evidence of a clean-based ulcer with a rebleeding risk of less than 5%. The appropriate course of action is to discontinue the NSAID and use a PPI to promote ulcer healing. A and B are not correct because you do not want to continue injury to the gastric mucosa. Choice C is not correct because the majority of clean-based ulcers will heal with therapy, and the likelihood of rebleeding from a clean-based ulcer is low.

36. **(D)** Oil mount is used to identify the *Sarcoptes scabiei* mite.

37. **(C)** In OSA, there is a significant increase in the resistance to airflow during inspiration, leading to apneas or hypopneas during sleep. Arousal is required to allow return of pharyngeal muscle tone and adequate flow of air. As a result, patients with OSA have severely fragmented sleep leading to their difficulties with daytime hypersomnolence. The hallmark of therapy for OSA is CPAP therapy. This provides an "air splint" to maintain patency of the upper airways, preventing collapse and therefore apneas. OSA can sometimes be positional, in which case position restriction may be helpful. As obesity is felt to contribute to the narrowing of the pharynx, weight loss should always be encouraged. Surgical options are available and are useful in select cases. Tracheostomy, for example, was the first effective treatment available for OSA. Other surgeries include attempts to remodel the upper airway to maintain its patency. The desaturations that occur due to OSA should not be treated with oxygen. The desaturations are a result of airflow obstruction and therefore treatment should be geared toward returning airflow. Therefore, if no underlying gas exchange abnormalities exist (as with emphysema), oxygen therapy is not necessary.

38. (C) This patient presents with gastrinoma resulting in gastric acid hypersecretion. Although rare in Zollinger-Ellison syndrome, there are several well-documented instances of jejunal ulcerations presenting as the first manifestation of this syndrome. *H. pylori* infection is not generally known to cause jejunal ulcerations. There is no history to suggest that the patient is immunocompromised; therefore, CMV infection is unlikely. Although potassium chloride has been shown to induce jejunal ulcerations, the patient denies taking medications.

39. (D) The diagnosis of MI is based on several features. Clinical symptoms and electrocardiographic (ECG) changes are corroborated by cardiac enzymes. Generally, CK rises within 6 to 8 hours after an MI and peaks in about 24 hours. Typically, by 48 to 96 hours the levels will have returned to baseline. Troponin I and T are more specific tests for myocardial damage. Troponin begins to rise within 3 hours of MI. LDH is less sensitive and the myocardial isoenzyme (LDH1) begins to rise 24 to 48 hours after an MI and peaks in 3 to 5 days. It will typically return to baseline in 7 to 10 days.

40. (C) A poorly differentiated carcinoma with evidence of stalk invasion would prompt a surgical referral for resection because of the high likelihood of extension through the lamina propria. Repeat colonoscopy would place the patient at risk for extension of the tumor. It would be premature without evidence of systemic spread of the tumor to warrant a referral to an oncologist.

41. (A) *V. cholera* leads to a protracted course of watery diarrhea, often leading to orthostatic hypotension. The patient was obviously visiting an area of the world where this organism is endemic. The absence of blood and the clinical scenario would go against a *C. difficile* infection. Rotavirus, although possible, would not generally lead to fever. Enterotoxigenic strains of *E. coli* are a result of consumption of foods that contain the preformed toxin, which leads to the symptoms of crampy abdominal pain and diarrhea but generally does not lead to fever and orthostatic hypotension.

42. (E) Emergency contraceptive (or "morning after") pills are initiated in the first 72 hours after a single act of unprotected intercourse and are very effective postcoital contraception. FDA-approved preparations in the United States contain either levonorgestrel alone or a combination of ethinyl estradiol and levonorgestrel. Misoprostol (a prostaglandin E1 analog) and RU 486 (an antiprogestational agent) are used in combination for medical, early first trimester, termination of pregnancy. Diethylstilbestrol, while used in earlier formulations of the "morning after pill" is no longer in use for this purpose. Prostaglandin E2 as a cervical ripening agent utilized prior to induction of labor.

43. (D) Administration of anti-D antibodies in the immediate postpartum period to an Rh-negative mom giving birth to an Rh-positive baby prevents most maternal Rh sensitization. Rh-sensitized mothers can have future pregnancies affected by fetal hemolytic anemia and immune hydrops and even fetal death. While maternal–fetal ABO incompatibility is a cause of usually milder neonatal jaundice when maternal blood type is O and the baby's is A, B, or AB, this is not preventable by administration of anti-D antibodies. Maternal rubella infection can be disastrous to the fetus early in pregnancy so nonimmune moms usually receive rubella immunization after delivery. Maternal chickenpox is less likely to cause neonatal abnormalities but when the mom has active disease at the time of delivery, infant exposure can lead to neonatal infection, which can be quite severe.

44. (C) The biceps femoris has two heads and functions as a hip flexor and a knee flexor. Its insertion is on the head of the fibula.

45. (C) Folic acid supplementation both prior to and in very early pregnancy greatly decreases the chance of all types of neural tube defects, including spina bifida. However, since these defects occur very early in the first trimester, initiating folic acid supplementation at 20 weeks would not affect her chance of having a baby with spina bifida. The chance of having a baby with a chromosomal disorders increases with maternal age, age is not a risk factor for having a baby with neural tube defects.

46. **(D)** Squamous cell carcinomas can secrete PTHrp, which, like PTH, causes hypercalcemia.

47. **(C)** Patients with multiple endocrine neoplasia type 1 (MEN 1) have four-gland hyperplasia. Patients with sporadic primary hyperparathyroidism will have a single adenoma most of the time. Parathyroid carcinoma and double adenomas are rare.

48. **(C)** There is no established safe level of alcohol intake in pregnancy. Fetal alcohol syndrome is the most frequently recognized cause of mental retardation in the United States. However, the recognizable syndrome of mental retardation, hyperactivity, early irritability followed by growth deficiency and developmental delay that characterizes fetal alcohol syndrome is most commonly seen in heavy drinkers of more that two drinks/day throughout pregnancy and in binge drinkers

who have more than four drinks on frequent occasions during pregnancy. Women who drink more than eight drinks/day have a 30% to 50% risk of giving birth to an affected child. Cessation of alcohol use early in pregnancy decreases risk considerably.

49. **(D)** Myocarditis is generally an acute or subacute illness that may give rise to chronic myocardial dysfunction. It is an inflammatory process involving the myocardium and may have a variety of causes. The most common cause in the United States is viral. It can range from an acute devastating illness with myocardial dysfunction to a subacute presentation wherein the patient presents for evaluation of the underlying infectious process. Pain, if present, tends to be atypical, but pleuritic or positional pain is associated with pericarditis, not myocarditis.

50. **(B)** Positional changes result in a variety of compensatory changes that facilitate maintenance of normal blood pressure in the upright position. These include enhanced vasomotor tone, which results primarily through sympathetic activation. Sympathetic activation enhances myocardial function. Drugs such as ganglionic blocking drugs can impair the autonomic reflex mechanism and result in or worsen orthostatis.

Practice Test 6
Questions

DIRECTIONS (Questions 1 through 50): Each of the numbered items or incomplete statements in this section is followed by answers or by completions of the statement. Select the ONE lettered heading or completion that is BEST in each case.

1. A patient is seen in the clinic. On physical exam, the following findings were noted: The left ventricular impulse feels hyperdynamic. A grade II/VI holosystolic murmur that is musical in quality is heard at the apex and radiates to the axilla. A third heart sound is present. The murmur increases with expiration. These findings are consistent with which of the following?

   (A) mitral regurgitation
   (B) tricuspid regurgitation
   (C) mitral valve prolapse (MVP)
   (D) innocent murmur
   (E) aortic stenosis

2. Which of the following preventable infectious diseases is still responsible for severe musculoskeletal deformities in children in many developing countries?

   (A) smallpox
   (B) poliomyelitis
   (C) tuberculosis
   (D) muscular dystrophy
   (E) varicella

3. A 60-year-old woman complains of pain and swelling of the right flank. Urinalysis reveals hematuria, and computed tomography (CT) shows a large, partially necrotic mass replacing the upper pole of the right kidney. What is the most likely lesion?

   (A) transitional cell cancer
   (B) tuberculosis
   (C) adrenal cortical adenoma
   (D) renal cell carcinoma
   (E) endometriosis

4. Which of the following is the causative organism of scabies infestations?

   (A) mite
   (B) louse
   (C) flea
   (D) bedbug
   (E) tick

5. A 1-week-old infant, delivered at home by a midwife, is brought to the hospital by his mother because she has noticed ecchymoses as well as some blood in the infant's stools. The prenatal course as well as the delivery went very well, and the infant is otherwise healthy. What is the likely explanation for the infant's bleeding difficulties?

   (A) vitamin A deficiency
   (B) vitamin A toxicity
   (C) vitamin B_{12} deficiency
   (D) vitamin C deficiency
   (E) vitamin K deficiency

6. The photomicrograph shown in Figure 6.1 is an example of which of the following?

(A) plasmacytoma
(B) giant cell tumor
(C) Ewing's sarcoma
(D) lymphoma
(E) leukemia

7. A patient is seen in the clinic. On physical exam, the following findings were noted: The neck veins were prominent. A grade III/VI late systolic murmur that increases with inspiration was present. The murmur was best heard along the left sternal border. These findings are consistent with

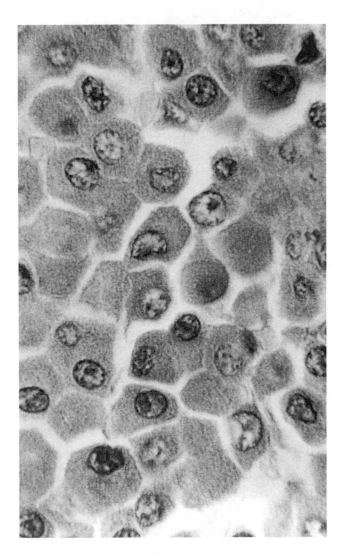

Figure 6.1

(A) mitral regurgitation
(B) tricuspid regurgitation
(C) MVP
(D) innocent murmur
(E) aortic stenosis

8. A 22-year-old pregnant woman in her second trimester presents to the emergency department (ED) with fever, chills, right flank pain, and hemorrhage. She has a history of renal stones with her last pregnancy. Her creatinine and urea nitrogen are 1.3 mg and 18, respectively. What are the most common changes in glomerular filtration rate (GFR) and renal plasma flow (RPF) during pregnancy?

(A) increased GFR and decreased RPF
(B) increased RPF and decreased GFR
(C) increased RPF and increased GFR
(D) decreased GFR and decreased RPF
(E) decreased GFR and increased PPF

9. A 53-year-old man is seen for osteomalacia due to vitamin D deficiency. Which of the following combinations of laboratory tests will he most likely have?

	Serum Calcium	Serum Phosphate	PTH
(A)	High	Low	High
(B)	Low	High	Normal
(C)	Low	Low	High
(D)	Low	High	Low
(E)	Normal	Normal	Low

10. In a patient with vitamin D deficiency, a characteristic finding on a pelvic x-ray would be

(A) sacroiliitis
(B) chondrocalcinosis
(C) Looser zones
(D) pectus excavatum
(E) pectus carinatum

11. Which of the following is true concerning pancreatic cancer?

(A) It never presents as acute pancreatitis.
(B) Jaundice is often present, especially in head-of-the-pancreas tumors.

(C) Back, midepigastric, and left upper quadrant pain are rare.

(D) Migratory thrombophlebitis or Trousseau's sign is atypical.

(E) It locally invades adjacent structures but rarely metastasizes distantly.

12. Hypertrophic cardiomyopathy (HCM)

(A) results from abnormal thickening of the pericardium and endocardium

(B) is associated with abnormal systolic but preserved diastolic function

(C) is in general an inherited disorder

(D) is associated with obstruction to left ventricular (LV) outflow at the aortic valve

(E) is easy to diagnose on physical exam

13. The cell type in the ovarian follicle responsible for the highest proportion of estrogen production is the

(A) theca cell

(B) granulosa cell

(C) oocyte

(D) lactotroph

(E) beta cell

Questions 14 through 16

Refer to Figure 6.2 for questions 14 through 16.

14. A 55-year-old patient presents with bitemporal hemianopsia. Where is the likely lesion along the optic pathways?

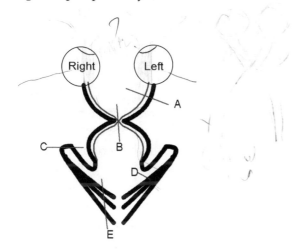

Figure 6.2

(A) A

(B) B

(C) C

(D) D

(E) E

15. A 65-year-old woman with a history of cerebrovascular disease presents with an acute loss of vision over her left visual field. Formal visual field testing reveals a left homonymous hemianopsia but with macular sparing. Where is the likely lesion?

(A) A

(B) B

(C) C

(D) D

(E) E

16. A 48-year-old man with acquired immune deficiency syndrome (AIDS) develops insidious loss of vision from his right eye. Gross visual testing confirms loss of vision in his right eye and preservation of vision in his left eye. Where is a magnetic resonance imaging (MRI) scan likely to identify a lesion?

(A) A

(B) B

(C) C

(D) D

(E) E

17. Which of the following conditions is associated with Crohn's disease:

(A) ankylosing spondylitis

(B) rheumatoid arthritis

(C) osteoarthritis

(D) Behçet's syndrome

(E) gouty arthritis

18. A 47-year-old patient presents with recurrence of pain following a lateral pancreaticojejunostomy (Puestow procedure). Your resident discusses the case with the patient's family, but one of his statements is inaccurate. Which one?

    (A) Pain may be from blockage of the secondary pancreatic ducts.
    (B) The patient may improve with endoscopic retrograde cholangiopancreatography (ERCP) to perform a sphincterotomy.
    (C) The patient may improve with a total pancreatectomy.
    (D) The pain may be due to an incomplete procedure's being performed.
    (E) The pain should be controlled.

19. You are evaluating a 40-year-old woman who underwent a laparoscopic cholecystectomy for acute cholecystitis 1 week ago. Postoperatively, the patient has complained of persistent nausea and abdominal distention. On examination the patient is afebrile. There is no scleral icterus, but there are diminished breath sounds over the right base of the lungs, and the abdomen is moderately distended with decreased bowel sounds. There is no rebound tenderness on the abdominal examination. Which of the following would be a possible cause of her symptoms?

    (A) bile leak following a bile duct injury
    (B) acute gastroenteritis
    (C) pseudomembranous colitis
    (D) gastroparesis
    (E) hepatitis

20. A 45-year-old man is admitted to the hospital with a chief complaint of vomiting, severe abdominal pain, and difficulty breathing. On examination the patient is mildly febrile and tachypneic, and on examination there is exquisite pain in the epigastrium. Which of the following should be evaluated for?

    (A) cecal diverticulitis
    (B) acute pancreatitis
    (C) gastroesophageal reflux disease (GERD)

    (D) pulmonary embolus
    (E) migraine

21. ERCP in the setting of biliary pancreatitis has been shown to result in which of the following?

    (A) should not be performed urgently
    (B) diagnose the presence of biliary stones
    (C) increase the need for urgent surgery
    (D) is generally performed with insertion of a biliary stent
    (E) death

22. Which of the following studies would be the most sensitive and specific for diagnosing a biliary etiology of acute pancreatitis?

    (A) elevated serum bilirubin
    (B) elevated serum amylase
    (C) elevated alkaline phosphatase
    (D) ultrasound evidence of a dilated common bile duct
    (E) elevated sedimentation rate

23. A 58-year-old woman has a T-score of −2.3 at the spine and −1.8 at the hip. What does she have?

    (A) osteoporosis at the spine and osteopenia at the hip
    (B) osteopenia at the spine and hip
    (C) osteoporosis at the spine and hip
    (D) osteopenia at the spine and osteoporosis at the hip
    (E) lab error

24. Regarding Eisenmenger syndrome, which of the following statements is correct?

    (A) In Eisenmenger syndrome, the pulmonary vasculature remains normal, but pulmonary pressures are elevated.
    (B) Pulmonary hypertension is severe and results in left-to-right shunting.
    (C) Eisenmenger syndrome can occur as a result of several types of lesions.
    (D) Eisenmenger syndrome is reversible in early stages.
    (E) Eisenmenger syndrome is reversible.

25. Which of the following is an etiology of tho-racolumbar scoliosis in female children?

    (A) cervical spinal cord injury
    (B) cerebral palsy
    (C) neurofibromatosis
    (D) Duchenne muscular dystrophy
    (E) hypothyroidism

26. The electrocardiogram (ECG) recording in Figure 6.3 was recorded in a patient known to be taking a medication. What drug is this patient likely taking?

    (A) procainamide hydrochloride
    (B) digoxin
    (C) captopril
    (D) flecainide
    (E) sildenafil

27. Myelomeningocele occurs due to an abnormality in which of the following embryonic stages or structures?

    (A) limb bud formation
    (B) neural tube closure
    (C) blastomere
    (D) mesoderm
    (E) mesothelium

28. The ECG recording in Figure 6.4 was recorded in a patient known to be taking a medication. What drug is this patient likely taking?

    (A) procainamide hydrochloride
    (B) digoxin
    (C) captopril
    (D) flecainide
    (E) merperidine

29. Syndactyly results from which of the following processes occurring in the limb bud before 8 weeks' gestation?

    (A) duplication
    (B) failure of formation
    (C) failure of programmed cell death
    (D) overgrowth
    (E) undergrowth

30. An asymmetry of vibration over both sides of the sternum, "give-away" weakness on motor testing, and a lack of concern about a severe physical "abnormality" may suggest an

    (A) psychosis
    (B) conversion disorder
    (C) impulse control disorder
    (D) learning disorder
    (E) normal reaction to disease

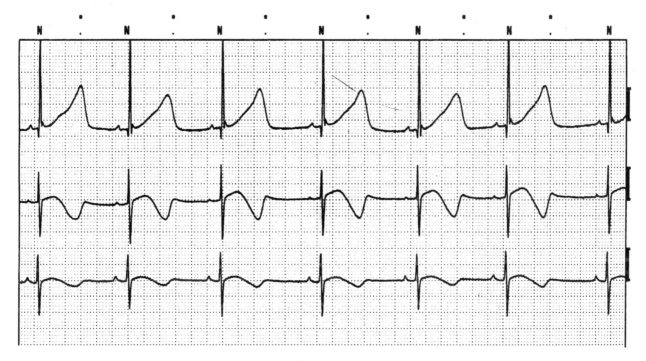

Figure 6.3

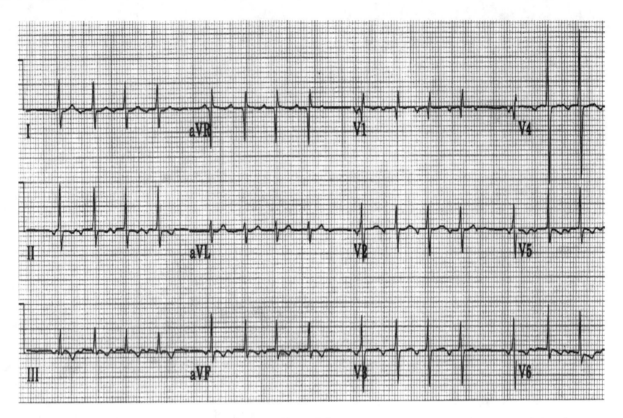

Figure 6.4

31. In which blood vessel is the partial pressure of oxygen (PO_2) the highest?

    (A) umbilical vein
    (B) umbilical artery
    (C) fetal pulmonary capillary
    (D) maternal endometrial vein
    (E) maternal hepatic veins

32. Which structure is a branch of the anterior hypogastric artery?

    (A) iliac artery
    (B) ureter
    (C) anterior hypogastric vein
    (D) posterior hypogastric artery
    (E) uterine artery

33. The genetic material found in a complete hydatidiform mole is

    (A) always aneuploid
    (B) of both maternal and paternal origin
    (C) of paternal origin only
    (D) of maternal origin only
    (E) of new origin

34. The preferred surgical management of a pleomorphic adenoma of the parotid gland is

    (A) radical parotidectomy
    (B) radical parotidectomy with neck dissection
    (C) simple enucleation of the tumor
    (D) superficial parotidectomy
    (E) superficial parotidectomy with lymph node dissection

35. A 44-year-old woman has Crohn's disease that has required multiple bowel surgeries. She presents to her primary care physician with a bony pain in her hips and lower extremities. She recalls no trauma. An x-ray is performed and Looser-Milkman pseudofractures are found, in addition to radiographic osteopenia. A bone densitometry is then performed, revealing advanced osteoporosis. What is the likely cause of this patient's premature osteoporosis?

(A) vitamin A deficiency

(B) vitamin A toxicity

(C) vitamin B$_{12}$ deficiency

(D) vitamin C deficiency

(E) vitamin D deficiency

36. A 48-year-old man with a long history of alcohol use was recently diagnosed with hepatitis C, and a liver biopsy revealed inflammation consistent with hepatitis C. The past history is otherwise noncontributory except that the patient has also been treated for bipolar disease by his psychiatrist. Which of the following would be the most appropriate management strategy?

(A) Initiate therapy with interferon in combination with ribavirin.

(B) Discontinue alcohol therapy and then start treatment with interferon in combination with ribavirin.

(C) Obtain psychiatric clearance for treatment with interferon and ribavirin following an alcohol cessation program for at least 6 months.

(D) Intitiate therapy with interferon alone.

(E) Avoid interferon in this case.

37. A 50-year-old woman with a history of watery diarrhea and an elevated gastrin level (fasting gastrin level = 2000 pg/mL; normal < 100 pg/mL) is being worked up. An endoscopic ultrasound examination shows a gastrinoma in the pancreatic body. Which of the following would be the most likely diagnosis?

(A) Zollinger-Ellison syndrome

(B) carcinoid syndrome

(C) multiple endocrine neoplasia type 2 (MEN 2)

(D) nonfunctional islet cell tumor

(E) irritable bowel syndrome

38. A 70-year-old man presents with left shoulder pain. On examination, he is found to have a barrel chest and diminished air movement. His cardiovascular examination is normal. His pupils are asymmetric with notable miosis of his left pupil. He had never noticed this himself. What initial test is likely to suggest the cause of this patient's shoulder pain?

(A) cardiac stress test

(B) chest x-ray

(C) shoulder films

(D) cervical spine films

(E) thyroid examination

39. Under which of the following conditions would you refer a patient with a long-standing history of reflux esophagitis for a Nissen fundoplication?

(A) a young patient with no other medical problems who responds favorably to proton pump inhibitors (PPIs)

(B) a young patient with no other medical problems who fails to respond to PPIs

(C) an elderly patient with multiple medical problems including an ejection fraction of less than 10% who has responded well to PPIs

(D) a patient who responds well to PPIs and has a diagnosis of scleroderma

(E) a young patient with scleroderma

40. The endoscopic picture in Figure 6.5 was obtained from the pylorus in a 45-year-old patient. What does the biopsy show?

(A) normal duodenal mucosa

(B) normal esophageal mucosa

(C) gastric mucosal hyperplasia

(D) colonic mucosa

(E) colonic polyps

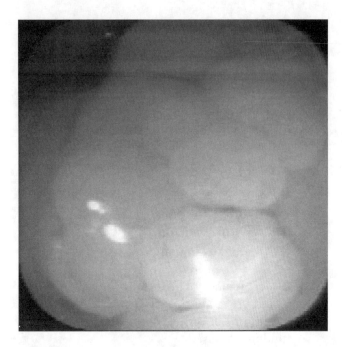

Figure 6.5

41. A 69-year-old obese woman presents with new-onset diplopia and pain over her left eye. Examination further reveals a mild ptosis of the left eye. Pupillary exam is unremarkable. Which test is likely to suggest a diagnosis that is the likely cause of this patient's diploplia?

(A) MRI of head to rule out compressive lesion of cranial nerve (CN) III
(B) thyroid examination and thyroid function tests
(C) fasting glucose
(D) chest CT with attention to the left superior sulcus
(E) lumbar puncture

42. A 67-year-old hypertensive man presents with the acute onset, just 1 hour prior to his arrival in the ED, of left-sided homonomous hemianopsia, left body neglect, and loss of graphesthesia in the left hand. He has no motor weakness. His blood pressure is 160/100 and his heart rate is 88 and regular. Routine lab work including platelet count and coagulation studies are normal. An urgent CT scan of the head is normal. What treatment should be given acutely in the ED?

(A) intravenous heparin
(B) low-molecular-weight heparin
(C) tissue plasminogen activator
(D) warfarin
(E) aspirin

43. Which muscle does the trochlear nerve innervate?

(A) lateral rectus
(B) inferior rectus
(C) superior rectus
(D) inferior oblique
(E) superior oblique

44. Progression of disability has been slowed by which of the following therapeutic agents used to treat multiple sclerosis (MS)?

(A) beta-interferon-1A
(B) beta-interferon-1B
(C) glatiramer acetate
(D) intravenous methylprednisolone
(E) oral prednisone

45. Which neurodegenerative disease is associated with the type IV allele of apolipoprotein E?

(A) Alzheimer's disease
(B) Pick's disease
(C) Parkinson's disease
(D) Wilson's disease
(E) amyotrophic lateral sclerosis

Questions 46 and 47

46. Which nerve arising from the brachial plexus does the suprascapular nerve supply?

(A) serratus anterior
(B) biceps
(C) brachioradialis
(D) infraspinatus
(E) deltoid

47. Which peripheral nerve arising from the brachial plexus does the musculocutaneous nerve supply?

    (A) serratus anterior
    (B) biceps
    (C) brachioradialis
    (D) infraspinatus
    (E) deltoid

48. A 26-year-old woman in the first trimester of her pregnancy presents with primary syphilis and has an allergy to penicillin. What is the treatment of choice?

    (A) erythromycin
    (B) doxycyline
    (C) ciprofloxacin
    (D) trimethoprim–sulfamethoxazole
    (E) desensitization followed by penicillin

49. A 42-year-old woman with urticaria is prescribed a combination of antihistamines. Which of the following has both H_1 and H_2 activity?

    (A) diphenhydramine
    (B) doxepin
    (C) hydroxyzine
    (D) loratadine
    (E) cyproheptadine

50. A 22-year-old woman newly diagnosed with a psychiatric condition presents with an abrupt worsening of her her acne, which had been well controlled with topical antibiotics. Which of the following is most likely one of her medications?

    (A) doxepin
    (B) lithium
    (C) sertraline
    (D) bupropion
    (E) gabapentin

Answers and Explanations

1. **(A)** The left ventricular impulse is often hyperdynamic owing to the excess blood volume. The murmur is holosystolic and increases on expiration. An S3 is often present. The murmur is present at the apex and radiates to the axilla.

2. **(B)** Poliomyelitis is still present in developing areas due to lack of vaccine. The poliovirus invades the body through the oropharyngeal route, multiplies in the lymph nodes of the alimentary tract, then spreads by the hematogenous route to the anterior horn cells of the spinal cord, producing paralysis. Paralysis can be transient depending on the extent of anterior horn cell damage and the ability of the cell bodies and axons to regenerate. A muscle still paralyzed at 6 months will remain so. Paralysis leads to muscle and joint contractures with severe deformities.

3. **(D)** Hematuria, pain, and a flank mass are characteristic symptoms of renal cell cancer. The CT presentation is also consistent with renal cell carcinoma. Renal cell cancers often hemorrhage and show necrosis.

4. **(A)** Scabies is caused by the mite *Sarcoptes scabiei.*

5. **(E)** Vitamin K deficiency is characterized by findings suggesting impaired coagulation such as easy bruisability, mucosal bleeding, splinter hemorrhages, melena, hematochezia, and hematuria. Vitamin K is a coenzyme in the carboxylation of glutamate to gamma-carboxyglutamate, which is a necessary component of clotting factors II, VII, IX, and X. It is also found in proteins C and S. The infant described likely has hemorrhagic disease of the newborn, which typically occurs 1 to 7 days postpartum. The vitamin deficiency in this setting may be due to an immature liver, low vitamin K content in breast milk, low transplacental transfer of vitamin K, and a sterile gut. Normal levels are found usually a month after birth. Manifestations include cutaneous, gastrointestinal, and sometimes intracranial bleeding. Risk factors may include certain antibiotics, anticonvulsants, and Coumadin ingestion. The current recommendations are to administer parenteral vitamin K at birth to all neonates, in addition to infant formula supplementation with vitamin K.

6. **(A)** All of the tumors are round-cell tumors with the exception of giant cell tumor. It is characterized by multinucleated giant cells on a benign background stroma. Plasmacytomas (multiple myeloma) contain sheets of plasma cells recognizable by their "clock face" nuclei. Bone lesions are lytic appearing and cause very little reactive bone formation, rendering them "cold" on bone scan.

7. **(B)** The murmur of tricuspid regurgitation can be quite variable. There can be an early systolic murmur and a holosystolic bruit or a bruit that ends at S2. The murmur is elicited by inspiration and is best heard at the left sternal border. Neck veins are typically elevated, and the liver is pulsatile in severe tricuspid regurgitation.

8. **(A)** Glomerular filtration rate (GFR) is increased in pregnancy. Renal plasma flow (RPF) is decreased.

9. **(C)** Patients with vitamin D deficiency have secondary hyperparathyroidism. Overall, calcium and phosphate will be low/normal with high PTH.

10. **(C)** In osteomalacia, Looser zones or pseudofractures are seen. Sacroiliitis is seen in ankylosing spondylitis. Pectus excavatum and carinatum are congenital. Chondrocalcinosis is the deposition of calcium crystals in the joints.

11. **(C)** When diagnosed, pancreatic cancer is either locally advanced or metastatic. Jaundice, back and abdominal pain, acute pancreatitis, and thrombophlebitis may be present in patients as well.

12. **(C)** HCM is a disease manifested by abnormal myocardial thickening. This can result in outflow obstruction below the level of the aortic valve. In some cases, no obstruction is present. Most patients with HCM have preserved LV systolic function but impaired diastolic relaxation. Later in the disease, systolic dysfunction can occur. It is inherited in over half the cases and multiple genotypes have been described.

13. **(B)** While theca cells have the ability to convert precursor androstenedione and testosterone to estrogens, the aromatose activity necessary for this conversion is much higher in granulosa cells. Oocytes are not thought to be responsible for significant hormonal production. Lactotrophs are the cells in the anterior pituitary responsible for prolactin secretion.

14. **(B)** The optic nerve from each eye meets at the optic chiasm and the fibers in the nasal ganglion cells cross to the contralateral side. These nasal ganglion cells transmit vision from the temporal fields. A midline lesion compressing at the optic chiasm such as with a pituitary adenoma, craniopharyngioma, meningioma, glioma, or an aneurysm will therefore result in a bitemporal hemianopsia. Bitemporal hemianopsia can develop insidiously and may be picked up only by an as- tute clinician or by formal testing of visual fields.

15. **(E)** Homonymous hemianopsia is loss of a visual field, and therefore by definition implicates involvement of both eyes. For this to be the case, the lesion or defect must be posterior to the optic chiasm. A lesion involving the entire optic tract anywhere posterior to the optic chiasm will cause a homonymous hemianopsia. Only E in the diagram shows complete transaction of the optic radiations posterior to the optic chiasm. Furthermore, sparing of the macula can occur following occlusion of the posterior cerebral artery, as the macular representation situated at the tip of the occipital lobes is supplied by collaterals from the middle cerebral arteries. This makes lesion E even more likely than any of the other choices.

16. **(A)** Loss of vision from an eye (versus loss of vision from a visual field) suggests a lesion anywhere anterior to the optic chiasm. This may be at the level of the lens or retina or involve the optic nerve. In a patient with AIDS, multiple entities are possible, including cytomegalovirus (CMV) retinitis, cerebral lymphoma, and toxoplasmosis.

17. **(A)** The extraintestinal complications of Crohn's disease and ulcerative colitis are generally related to inflammatory disease activity These complications, which tend to be more frequent with colonic involvement, include uveitis and episcleritis, and skin disorders such as erythema nodosum and pyoderma gangrenosum. Another extraintestinal manifestation includes peripheral arthritis, which primarily involves large joints (with no synovial destruction), and ankylosing spondylitis. Ankylosing spondylitis may be the presenting manifestation of Crohn's disease. Rheumatoid arthritis and osteoarthritis, which involve synovial destruction, are not associated with inflammatory bowel disease.

18. **(C)** Pain following this procedure is most commonly due to either an incomplete procedure's being performed or blockage of the

secondary pancreatic radicles. A drainage procedure such as that which can be performed using a sphincterotomy may improve the symptoms. A complete pancreatectomy would certainly solve the problem but with a great deal of morbidity.

19. **(A)** Following a cholecystectomy performed laparoscopically, the most common cause for postoperative complication is a bile leak caused by incomplete closure of the bile duct. The other options listed would be uncommon causes of morbidity following this procedure.

20. **(B)** The patient in question is more likely to have a case of acute pancreatitis. Cecal diverticulitis may be associated with abdominal pain or bleeding but does not generally result in epigastric pain. GERD could result in epigastric pain but will not cause fever or tachypnea.

21. **(B)** ERCP can be performed urgently in the setting of an acute biliary pancreatitis to identify and extract a bile duct stone. ERCP in this setting would therefore decrease the need for an urgent operation, and in most cases does not require the insertion of a biliary stent.

22. **(D)** An elevation in the serum bilirubin, amylase, or alkaline phosphatase lack specificity in the identification of a biliary source of pancreatitis. Ultrasound evidence of a dilated common bile duct would therefore be the most sensitive and specific modality listed.

23. **(B)** A T-score of < –2.5 defines osteoporosis. A T-score between –2.5 and –1 defines osteopenia.

24. **(C)** Eisenmenger syndrome refers to an irreversible condition where severe pulmonary hypertension has resulted in obliterative pulmonary vascular disease. It occurs in congenital lesions that cause severe enough pulmonary hypertension to result in reversal of flow with right-to-left shunting and resultant cyanosis.

25. **(D)** Duchenne muscular dystrophy is inherited as a sex-linked recessive illness. The ability to walk is lost by age 12 to 14. Once children become wheelchair bound, up to 80% develop an extreme collapsing scoliosis.

26. **(A)** Procainamide is a class Ia antiarrhythmic that can be used to treat atrial or ventricular arrhythmias. It suppresses phase 4 depolarization in normal ventricular muscle and Purkinje fibers. It reduces the automaticity of ectopic pacemakers. Procainamide is useful in treatment of reentry since it slows intraventricular conduction. Because of its electrophysiologic effect, it prolongs the QT interval and may put the patient at risk for torsades de pointes.

27. **(B)** Myelomeningocele occurs due to a failure of neural tube closure. The degree of involvement is related to the length of the neural tube that remains open. The neural tube closes from a cervical to sacral direction. The open neural tube is covered surgically shortly after birth, and a cerebrospinal fluid (CSF) shunt procedure is generally required. Children with only sacral involvement are ambulatory.

28. **(B)** This tracing shows paroxysmal atrial tachycardia (PAT) with block. This rhythm has been associated with digoxin, which is a cardiac glycoside. This drug has both direct and indirect effects on the heart. The direct effects are associated with its positive chronotropy. The indirect effects are mediated through the autonomic nervous system. The autonomic effects are vagomimetic and explain the slowing of the conduction at the atrioventricular (AV) node. At high doses a sympathomimetic effect may occur. Toxicity is often manifested by nausea, vomiting, anorexia, and diarrhea. A variety of abnormal rhythms, including PAT with block and ventricular tachycardia, are seen with digitalis toxicity.

29. **(C)** Failure of programmed cell death results in syndactyly of the fingers and toes. Syndactyly can be simple, involving only

skin and subcutaneous tissue, or complex, involving bone also.

30. **(B)** Conversion disorder is often part of a larger somatoform disorder in which an underlying psychiatric condition is present and there is a subconscious secondary gain. The much less common malingering involves a primary gain. The lack of concern over physical defects is also called *la belle indifference.* Before making a diagnosis of conversion disorder, all "organic" disorders must be excluded by extensive neurodiagnostic testing.

31. **(A)** The umbilical veins carry oxygenated fetal blood away from the fetal side of the placental villi to the fetus. The umbilical artery returns deoxygenated blood from the fetus to the villi. Fetal pulmonary capillary PO_2 would be lower than umbilical vein PO_2 since the fetus gets oxygen from the placental circulation and not the fetal lungs. Maternal endometrial veins take deoxygenated maternal blood away from the maternal side of the placenta.

32. **(C)** The iliac artery comes off the aorta and then branches to form the anterior and posterior hypogastric arteries. The uterine artery, which courses under the ureter, is a branch of the anterior hypogastric artery.

33. **(C)** Complete hydatidiform moles have no identifiable fetal tissue. Chromosomal analysis is most often 46XX and all chromosomes are of paternal origin.

34. **(D)** A pleomorphic adenoma of the parotid gland is considered a benign tumor, and thus neck dissection is unnecessary. This is usually found in the superficial lobe of the parotid gland near the seventh cranial nerve. Usually, they are well circumscribed, but satellite nodules may project from the tumor. Thus, shelling out the tumor or simple enucleation is not sufficient since recurrence can be high from any remaining tissue.

35. **(E)** This patient likely has osteomalacia. Crohn's disease is frequently associated with corticosteroid use and in of itself can lead to

premature osteoporosis. Another potential mechanism, however, in this patient is that she is malabsorbing vitamin D and/or calcium as a result of her inflammatory bowel disease and its complications. In particular, as vitamin D is fat soluble, its absorption may be hindered by steatorrhea, which can be common in patients with Crohn's disease. The deficiency in vitamin D can lead to bone remodeling and demineralization. Pathologic fractures, osteopenia, and incomplete ribbon-like areas of demineralization (called Looser's lines) can be seen on x-rays. Vitamin D deficiency can also occur as a result of low dietary intake, inadequate sunlight exposure, pancreatic insufficiency, small-bowel disease, malabsorption, postgastrectomy, diminished calcidiol production as in patients with liver disease, and decreased renal production of calcitriol as in patients with renal failure.

36. **(C)** Patients with hepatitis C and a history of alcohol use should be enrolled in an alchohol cessation program and remain abstinent for at least 6 months prior to treatment with interferon and ribavirin. Patients with a history of psychiatric illness should be cleared by a psychiatrist prior to initiating therapy for the hepatitis C because of the possible induction of suicidal tendency.

37. **(A)** Zollinger-Ellison syndrome is established as a diagnosis by the presence of an elevated serum gastrin level in the presence of gastric acid hypersecretion. The endoscopic ultrasound shows the gastrinoma in the pancreatic body. Carcinoid syndrome would cause diarrhea but is not associated with an elevated serum gastrin, and the tumor is generally in the bowel wall. MEN 2 refers to the presence of tumors involving the adrenal glands and not the pancreas. MEN 1, on the other hand, can be associated in up to one third of cases of Zollinger-Ellison syndrome. A nonfunctional islet cell tumor would not be associated with an elevation in serum hormone level.

38. **(B)** Horner syndrome is characterized by unilateral miosis, anhidrosis, and ptosis. This suggests disruption of the sympathetic out-

flow from the ipsilateral paravertebral sympathetic chain and the stellate (inferior cervical) ganglion. In a patient with likely emphysema from prior smoking and with shoulder pain, a superior sulcus (Pancoast) tumor compressing on the stellate ganglion on the ipsilateral side must be considered. A chest x-ray is therefore the best initial test. Pancoast tumors are usually bronchogenic and are associated with Horner syndrome in 14% to 50%. Other neurologic complications may occur with invasion of the tumor into the nerve roots, manifesting with weakness, muscle atrophy, and/or paresthesias involving the arm. Pain occurs from local invasion, including into the brachial plexus, and may radiate.

39. **(A)**   In general, patients who respond favorably to medical management of GERD should be considered for surgical therapy. If a patient fails medical management, you should consider an alternative diagnosis. Patients who have been diagnosed with other conditions such as scleroderma may not respond favorably to a Nissen fundoplication.

40. **(C)**   The pylorus normally contains gastric mucosa and not duodenal, esophageal, or colonic mucosa. In this particular biopsy the patient was noted to have hyperplasia of the gastric glands.

41. **(C)**   Although symmetric polyneuropathy is the most common neuropathic manifestation of diabetes, mononeuropathies can also occur. The most common cranial mononeuropathy due to diabetes involves the nerves supplying the extraocular muscles. Presentation may suggest dysfunction of cranial nerve III, IV, or VI but with normal pupillary function. A compressive lesion typically affects the parasympathetic fibers of CN III first, causing pupillary dysfunction.

42. **(C)**   When administered within the first 3 hours after an acute stroke, tissue plasminogen activator has been shown to reduce the eventual disability. There have been no studies proving any acute benefit to stroke outcome for the other therapies listed.

43. **(E)**   The lateral rectus is innervated by the abducens nerve (CN VI). The other muscles are innervated by the oculomotor nerve (CN III).

44. **(A)**   Only beta-interferon-1A has been able to show slowing of disability in MS patients. Beta-interferon-1B and glatiramer acetate, long with beta-interferon-1A, have shown benefit in decreasing relapse rate and improving MRI findings. Intravenous methylprednisolone may be useful in shortening the duration and lessening the severity of clinical exacerbations.

45. **(A)**   Two copies of the allele seem to impose a higher risk, but normal individuals can have the allele without developing the disease. Amyloid deposition in neuritic plaques and blood vessels has been correlated with whether there are one or two copies of the apo E type IV allele. Apo E is also found in neurofibrillary tangles.

46–47. **(46-D, 47-B)**   The brachial plexus may be affected by stretch injuries and is prone to iatrogenic radiation damage in the setting of breast cancer with axillary lymph node spread. Idiopathic brachial neuritis (Parsonnage-Turner syndrome) is an autoimmune condition occurring after recent infection, trauma, or remote surgery and is associated with deep, aching pain followed by rapid weakness and atrophy. The prognosis in idiopathic brachial neuritis is excellent, with full recovery of muscle function seen in 80% of patients by 1 year after onset.

48. **(E)**   Pregnant patients with syphilis who have a penicillin allergy should be desensitized and treated with the appropriate penicillin regimen.

49. **(B)**   Doxepin is a tricyclic antidepressant with H_1 and H_2 antihistamine activity. All of the other drugs listed are H_1 antihistamines.

50. **(B)**   Lithium can make existing skin conditions such as acne and psoriasis worse.

Practice Test 7
Questions

DIRECTIONS (Questions 1 through 50): Each of the numbered items or incomplete statements in this section is followed by answers or by completions of the statement. Select the ONE answer or completion that is BEST in each case.

1. A 48-year-old woman presents with a prolonged QT interval on her electrocardiogram (ECG). She has no symptoms and no family history of sudden cardiac death. She is on no medications. Which of the following statements is correct?

    (A) Her prognosis is excellent and she needs take no precautions.
    (B) She should be counseled to avoid certain medications including potassium-wasting diuretics.
    (C) Her prognosis is poor and she should have an implantable cardioverter defibrillator (ICD) implanted.
    (D) She is likely suffering from a congenital abnormality that affects the calcium channels.
    (E) This condition should be treated with medication.

2. You decide to treat a patient with osteoporosis. You explain to her that the drug you want to give her can give esophagitis as a side effect. What is the drug?

    (A) estrogen
    (B) raloxifene
    (C) calcitonin
    (D) risedronate
    (E) calcium

3. A 65-year-old woman has extensive Paget's disease of bone. As a result of her disease, she is at risk of developing which of the following heart conditions?

    (A) coronary heart disease
    (B) coarctation of the aorta
    (C) mitral stenosis
    (D) congestive heart failure (CHF)
    (E) aortic regurgitation

4. A Chiari type I malformation is associated with

    (A) tiredness
    (B) meningomyelocele
    (C) protrusion of cerebellar tonsils through the foramen magnum
    (D) paresis
    (E) weakness

5. Carpal tunnel syndrome is an entrapment neuropathy of which nerve?

    (A) superficial radial nerve
    (B) lateral antebrachial cutaneous nerve
    (C) posterior interosseous nerve
    (D) ulnar nerve
    (E) median nerve

6. A 37-year-old woman is seen for intermittent, short episodes of chest pain that wake her up at night. Heart function is normal by echocardiogram and no ischemia is seen on a stress test. An episode of pain is witnessed in the hospital and is associated with ST segment elevation on her ECG. Which drug would be appropriate therapy?

    (A) digoxin
    (B) clonidine
    (C) nifedipine
    (D) propranolol
    (E) lisinopril

7. A patient read on the Internet that she might be at risk of developing a rare cancer as a result of her Paget's. Which of the following is she referring to?

    (A) Burkitt's lymphoma
    (B) chondrosarcoma
    (C) fibrosarcoma
    (D) osteosarcoma
    (E) angiosarcoma

8. A woman presents with bloody discharge from a nipple. What is the most likely diagnosis?

    (A) Paget's disease of the nipple
    (B) intraductal carcinoma
    (C) medullary carcinoma
    (D) mucinous carcinoma
    (E) intraductal papilloma

9. A patient tells you that she comes from a family with Lynch syndrome, type II variant. Given this family history, what gynecological cancer is she at most risk of developing?

    (A) cervical
    (B) vulvar
    (C) fallopian tube
    (D) endometrial
    (E) vaginal

10. A 60-year-old man with coronary heart disease that is stable and hypertension has an ejection fraction of 37%. He is admitted with

CHF after his blood pressure medications were increased. Which of his medications is most likely at fault?

    (A) isosorbide dinitrate 40 mg bid
    (B) ramipril 10 mg qd
    (C) dyazide 37.5/25 mg qd
    (D) tenormin 100 mg qd
    (E) aspirin 81 mg qd

11. A 58-year-old man with a history of hepatitis C infection and chronic alcohol abuse presents to the emergency department with abdominal pain, nausea, and vomiting. The patient admits to using approximately 6 grams per day of acetaminophen for chronic back pain. The physical examination reveals mild hypotension and right upper quadrant abdominal pain. The aspartate transaminase (AST) and alanine transaminase (ALT) are markedly elevated in the thousand range. Which of the following is the most likely diagnosis?

    (A) acetaminophen-induced hepatotoxicity
    (B) acute hepatitis C flare
    (C) alcoholic hepatitis
    (D) shock liver
    (E) hepatorenal syndrome

12. Figure 7.1 depicts the cardiac cycle. Which period as described below is systole?

    (A) the period from the beginning of section B through the end of section D
    (B) the period from the beginning of section E to the end of section A

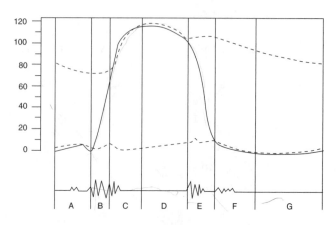

Figure 7.1

(C) A through E

(D) A through F

(E) A through B

13. A 21-year-old man developed right lower quadrant pain. He was found to have a pelvic kidney during the evaluation for the possible diagnosis of appendicitis. What vascular structures impeded the ascent of the right kidney?

(A) inferior mesenteric artery

(B) right common iliac artery

(C) right gondal artery

(D) right renal artery

(E) umbilical arteries

14. Intoxication with which of the following agents will commonly cause a seizure?

(A) diazepam

(B) lysergic acid diethylamide (LSD)

(C) model airplane glue (n-hexane)

(D) cocaine

(E) heroin

15. A 45-year-old man with a long history of alcohol abuse presents with acute onset of abdominal pain, nausea, and vomiting. Laboratory examination reveals elevation in the serum amylase and lipase consistent with acute pancreatitis. The patient is admitted to the hospital to receive intravenous fluids and is placed NPO. A computed tomographic (CT) examination of the abdomen reveals a cystic fluid collection in the pancreas. The most likely diagnosis of the condition is

(A) pancreatic adenocarcinoma

(B) pancreatic divisum

(C) obstruction of the common bile duct

(D) pseudocyst

(E) pancreatitis and hepatitis

16. A patient is taking medication for hypertension. He is asymptomatic and his blood pressure is well controlled. An ECG recording is obtained (see Figure 7.2). What should be done with his medications?

(A) maintain the current dose

(B) discontinue

(C) decrease the dose

(D) increase the dose

(E) add another medication

17. A young woman with paroxysmal supraventricular tachycardia (SVT) is seen in the ED for dizziness. She takes a medication for her arrhythmia and thinks she may have mistakenly taken a double dose. An ECG recording is obtained (Figure 7.3). What medication is she likely taking?

(A) nicardipine

(B) diltiazem

(C) quinidine

(D) mexiletine

(E) clonidine

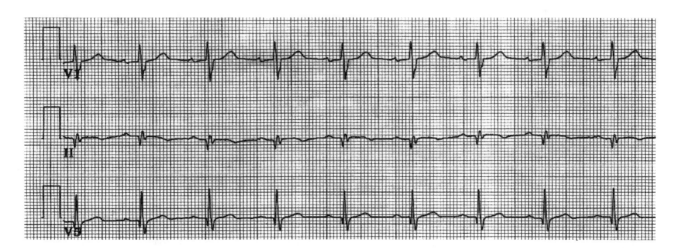

Figure 7.2

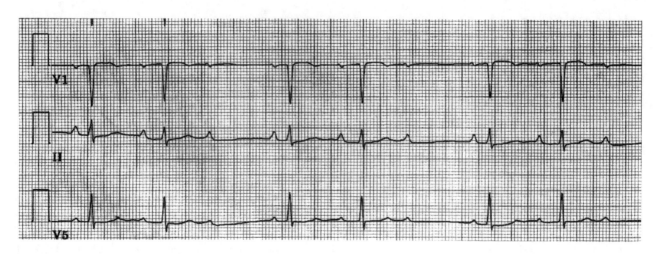

Figure 7.3

18. In the most recent studies in the United States the maternal mortality ratio was approximately

    (A) 1 maternal death/100 live births
    (B) 7 maternal deaths/100,000 live births
    (C) 18 maternal deaths/10,000 live births
    (D) 26 maternal deaths/100,000 live and stillbirths

19. A 60-year-old man with a history of small cell lung cancer develops weakness, hypertension, and hyperglycemia. An extensive evaluation concludes with a diagnosis of ectopic adrenocorticotropic hormone (ACTH) secretion by his lung cancer. Which of the following findings is consistent with this diagnosis?

    (A) hyperpigmentation
    (B) decreased ACTH secretion by the pituitary gland
    (C) suppression of cortisol levels by a high dose of dexamethasone
    (D) suppression of cortisol levels by a low dose of dexamethasone
    (E) anemia

20. Which of the following tumors is associated with occupational exposure to asbestos?

    (A) oat cell or small cell lung cancer
    (B) mesothelioma
    (C) squamous cell carcinoma
    (D) adenocarcinoma
    (E) bronchioalveolar carcinoma

21. The sun protection factor (SPF) refers to protection against which wavelength of light?

    (A) ultraviolet A
    (B) ultraviolet B
    (C) ultraviolet C
    (D) visible
    (E) infrared

22. A 47-year-old man is prescribed silbutramine for obesity after having failed multiple diet and exercise regimens. Which of the following best describes silbutramine's mechanism of weight reduction?

    (A) binds to intestinal fat
    (B) increases energy expenditure
    (C) suppresses appetite
    (D) inhibits growth of adipocytes
    (E) increases leptin levels

23. A 73-year-old institutionalized woman is brought by her daughter for a routine history and physical. She is noted to have a neuropathy, worse in her legs as compared to her arms. In particular, her vibration and position senses are impaired, and her shuffling gait is broad based. She had been complain-

ing of paresthesias, weakness, and fatigue as well. Her blood studies reveal a macrocytic anemia. What is the likely cause of the patient's neuropathy?

(A) vitamin A deficiency

(B) vitamin A toxicity

(C) vitamin B_{12} deficiency

(D) vitamin C deficiency

(E) folate deficiency

24. A serum alpha-fetoprotein and abdominal ultrasonography should be performed regularly in which of the following patients for the detection of hepatocellular carcinoma?

(A) patient with a history of smoking and excessive alcohol use

(B) patient with a diagnosis of hepatitis C and biopsy evidence of early cirrhosis

(C) patient with a positive hepatitis B surface antibody and negative surface antigen

(D) patient with a diagnosis of hepatitis A

(E) patient with strong family history

25. A 16-year-old girl presents with abdominal pain, amenorrhea, and vaginal bleeding. A pelvic examination reveals a left adnexal mass and uterine enlargement. Which of the following factors is unimportant with respect to ectopic pregnancy?

(A) prior tubal surgery

(B) in utero exposure to diethylstilbestrol (DES)

(C) prior history of pelvic inflammatory disease

(D) oral contraceptive use

(E) multiple sexual partners

26. Cholestasis has been associated with which of the following medications?

(A) penicillin G

(B) quinidine

(C) chlorpromazine

(D) 5-fluorouracil

(E) temazepam

27. Infants with colic typically cry

(A) rarely

(B) more than 3 hours per day, 3 days or more a week, for 3 or more weeks

(C) more than 10 minutes, twice a day

(D) 24 hours straight, once a week

(E) if not held

28. The most commonly isolated organism in adult osteomyelitis is

(A) *Staphylococcus aureus*

(B) *Escherichia coli*

(C) *Haemophilus influenzae*

(D) *Streptococcus pyogenes*

(E) *Mycobacterium tuberculosis*

29. Avascular necrosis (AVN) can affect which of the following bones?

(A) femoral head

(B) humeral shaft

(C) lateral femoral condyle

(D) capitate

(E) hallux metatarsal head

30. Which of the following germ cell tumors is the most common malignant tumor of the anterior mediastinum?

(A) choriocarcinoma

(B) seminoma

(C) endodermal sinus tumor

(D) embryonal cell carcinoma

(E) cystic teratoma

31. Which of the following is the causative agent of oral hairy leukoplakia?

(A) human herpesvirus type 8

(B) parvovirus

(C) poxvirus

(D) coxsackievirus

(E) Epstein-Barr virus

32. A 20-year-old college student presents to your office with a chief complaint of dysphagia. The patient is otherwise healthy and denies foreign travel. The patient is a nonsmoker and drinks alcohol occasionally with friends. As part of the workup you order a barium esophagram, which discloses a "bird beak appearance of the lower esophagus consistent with achalasia." Which of the following conditions best characterizes the physiology of achalasia?

(A) malignancy involving the esophagogastric junction

(B) normal esophageal motility and a significantly elevated lower esophageal sphincter (LES) pressure

(C) abnormal or absent motility in the esophagus and an elevated LES sphincter pressure

(D) significantly reduced LES pressure

(E) intermittent spasm

33. Which of the following is the most common type of breast carcinoma?

(A) medullary

(B) papillary

(C) mucinous

(D) infiltrating ductal

(E) intraductal

34. A loss of a normal ankle jerk during a neurologic exam indicates dysfunction of which nerve root?

(A) L3

(B) S1

(C) L4

(D) S2

(E) L5

35. Which of the following would be a poor initial step in the investigation of a patient with syncope?

(A) history

(B) physical

(C) ECG

(D) social history

(E) CT of the head

Questions 36 and 37

Questions 36 and 37 refer to the pathologic specimen shown in Figure 7.4.

36. The rapid passage of excitation through this structure is called

(A) membrane transport

(B) saltatory conduction

(C) axon transport

(D) excitation coupling

(E) receptor activation

37. Which channel is most numerous at the structure indicated by the arrow?

(A) sodium

(B) potassium

(C) chloride

(D) calcium

(E) magnesium

38. Which of the following statements is true regarding both the follicular cells and parafollicular C cells of the thyroid gland?

(A) Both produce calcitonin.

(B) Both produce thyroglobulin.

(C) Both reach the basement membrane of the thyroid follicle.

(D) Both are regulated by thyroid-stimulating hormone (TSH).

(E) Both are derived from the ultimobranchial body.

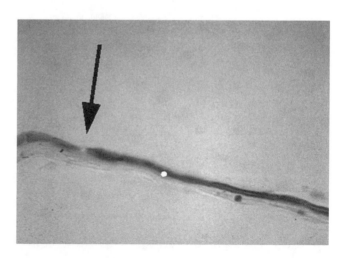

Figure 7.4

39. Which of the following would constitute alarm symptoms in a patient with a suspected diagnosis of functional bowel syndrome (irritable bowel syndrome)?

(A) weight loss
(B) diarrhea alternating with constipation
(C) pain on defecation
(D) bloating
(E) fever

40. A 62-year-old man recently completed chemotherapy with mitomycin and 5-fluorouracil for anal cell carcinoma. He was then found to have a hemoglobin of 9.0 g/dL and a platelet count of 66,000/μL and a peripheral smear was obtained. His smear is shown in Figure 7.5. The most likely diagnosis is

(A) iron deficiency
(B) hereditary spherocytosis
(C) myelofibrosis
(D) hemolytic–uremic syndrome
(E) vitamin B_{12} deficiency

41. Which of the following statements is innacurate regarding the development of the thyroid gland?

(A) The thyroid is the first endocrine gland to appear in embryonic development.
(B) Early in its development, the thyroid is connected to the tongue.
(C) The foramen cecum is the opening of the thyroglossal duct.

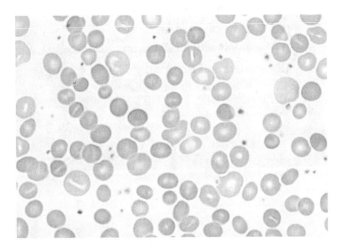

Figure 7.5

(D) The thyroglossal duct is normally present at birth and degenerates shortly after.
(E) The thyroid gland is derived from endodermal cells.

42. Your resident is discussing coronary artery bypass grafting (CABG) with a patient's family and you overhear him make four statements. Which statement would prompt you to interrupt and correct him?

(A) CABG involves using either arterial or venous conduits to bypass diseased sections of native coronary arteries.
(B) CABG is equal to medical therapy in relief of angina.
(C) Major complications of CABG include wound infection, perioperative myocardial infarction (MI), and bleeding.
(D) CABG improves survival in patients at moderate to high risk for medical therapy.
(E) CABG can be very effective in treatment of multivessel disease.

43. Which of the following has been implicated in the pathogenesis of Kaposi's sarcoma?

(A) human herpesvirus type 8
(B) parvovirus
(C) poxvirus
(D) coxsackievirus
(E) hepatitis C virus

44. A 23-year-old man is unresponsive due to severe head trauma following a motor vehicle accident. While in the intensive care unit, he develops significant polyuria and hypernatremia that is uncorrected by cessation of intravenous fluids. His glucose is normal. A urine osmolality is 100 mOsm/L, and a simultaneous serum osmolality is 330 mOsm/L. The attending decides to administer 10 μg of DDAVP (vasopressin) intranasally. A repeat measurement of the urine osmolality reveals 400 mOsm/L. What is the likely cause of the patient's polyuria?

(A) central diabetes insipidus (DI)
(B) nephrogenic polydipsia
(C) psychogenic polydipsia
(D) syndrome of inappropriate antidiuretic hormone (SIADH)
(E) diabetes mellitus (DM)

45. A patient develops acute respiratory distress syndrome (ARDS) as a complication of pancreatitis. The patient is electively intubated, and volume-controlled mechanical ventilatory support is initiated. The patient is 70 kg with a body mass index of 25 kg/m^2. The patient is initated on a low tidal-volume strategy on the ventilator with a tidal volume of 6 mL/kg of ideal body weight. However, the patient remains hypoxic on 80% Fio_2. Which of the following is likely to improve the patient's oxygenation?

(A) supine positioning

(B) nitric oxide

(C) decreasing positive end-expiratory pressure (PEEP)

(D) decreasing the Fio_2

(E) systemic corticosteroid

46. B-type natriuretic peptide (BNP) is likely to be elevated in which of the following conditions?

(A) HIV

(B) acute MI

(C) measles

(D) chronic cough of unknown etiology

(E) pneumonia

47. A patient develops progressive dyspnea 2 years out from his bilateral lung transplantation. Serial spirometry shows an obstructive ventilatory defect with steady decline in forced expiratory volume in 1 second (FEV_1). CT of the chest reveals a mosaic pattern. What is the likely diagnosis?

(A) bronchiolitis obliterans (BO) or constrictive bronchiolitis (CB)

(B) bronchiolitis obliterans with organizing pneumonia (BOOP) or cryptogenic organizing pneumonia (COP)

(C) invasive aspergillus

(D) cytomegalovirus (CMV) pneumonia

(E) particulate inhalation

48. A 54-year-old man with bronchiectasis presents to the ED with several episodes of brisk hemoptysis in the past 2 days. Embolization therapy is considered. Embolization of which vascular structure is likely to provide relief?

(A) pulmonary artery

(B) azygos vein

(C) bronchial artery

(D) internal mammary artery

(E) abdominal aorta

49. Which of the following hereditary diseases is associated with a trinucleotide repeat within the affected chromosome?

(A) Charcot-Marie-Tooth disease

(B) Duchenne's muscular dystrophy

(C) spinocerebellar degeneration

(D) MS

(E) myotonic dystrophy

50. A 23-year-old female medical student decides to begin jogging. She begins to note proximal muscle cramps and weakness after exercise. She had noticed no symptoms when running the 100-meter dash for her college track team. Exam revealed her to be of short stature with proximal muscle weakness. Ophthalmologic exam revealed early signs of retinitis pigmentosa. She admits that both her mother and maternal grandmother developed similar symptoms. What is the most likely diagnosis?

(A) glycogen storage disorder

(B) lipid storage disorder

(C) mucopolysaccharidosis

(D) mitochondrial disorder

(E) congenital myopathy

Answers and Explanations

1. **(B)** The patient likely has some form of long QT syndrome but is without features such as family history of sudden death or personal history of syncope that would confer a poor prognosis. Nonetheless, she should be cautioned to avoid drugs that prolong the QT interval further. The long QT syndromes have a variety of genetic bases involving the potassium and sodium channels.

2. **(D)** Bisphosphonates such as alendronate and risedronate can cause esophagitis.

3. **(D)** High-output CHF is a complication of Paget's disease.

4. **(C)** Meningomyelocele is frequently associated with a type II Chiari malformation. Clinical manifestations are infrequent but when present include ataxia, headache, and paralysis of the lower cranial nerves. More recent associations with generalized fatigue, peripheral pain, and syncope remain to be proven.

5. **(E)** The median nerve provides sensation to the thumb, index, long, and the radial half of the ring finger. Compression of this nerve by the transverse carpal ligament, which forms the roof of the carpal tunnel, produces this syndrome often seen as a result of repetitive motion in the workplace.

6. **(C)** This patient is most likely suffering from transient episodes of coronary vasospasm. The spasm can be treated or prevented by coronary vasodilators like nitrates or calcium channel blockers. Nifedipine is a potent vasodilator. While effective for other forms of angina, propranolol does not relax coronary artery smooth muscle. The other options play no role in coronary vasospasm.

7. **(D)** Though not common, osteosarcoma is a complication of Paget's disease.

8. **(E)** Nipple discharge is actually encountered more in benign conditions than in malignant tumors. Intraductal papilloma is the most common etiology. Papilloma is a discrete tumor of the connective tissue, and minor trauma to this layer may cause intermittent serous or serosanguineous discharge through the nipple.

9. **(D)** Lynch syndrome is synonymous with hereditary nonpolyposis colorectal cancer (HNPCC) and describes an autosomal-dominant tendency to develop colon cancer. Further subdivision is based on the familial presence of extracolon malignancies. Lynch type II has an association with endometrial cancer as well as other nongynecologic cancers.

10. **(D)** Tenormin is a beta blocker that is very effective for both hypertension and angina. It does, however, depress myocardial function and can decrease cardiac output, particularly in patients with left ventricular (LV) dysfunction. Ramipril, a tissue-specific angiotensin-converting enzyme (ACE) inhibitor will improve depressed function. Nitrates and diuretics have no direct impact on LV function but may be of benefit in depressed function by reducing LV preload.

11. **(A)** This case represents a classic example of acute hepatotoxicity resulting from excessive use of acetaminophen. Features suggesting acetaminophen toxicity include lack of illness prior to ingesting the drug, excessive use of acetaminophen, and concomitant use of alcohol. Hepatitis C generally does not result in a flare reaction. Acute hepatitis resulting from alcohol use does not result in high levels of AST and ALT. Shock liver can result in transaminase elevations in the thousand range, but there is no history in the case of acute hypotension.

12. **(A)** Systole is present from the beginning of section B through the end of section D. Ventricular pressure starts to rise rapidly almost immediately after the QRS complex is inscribed and systole has begun. The increase in ventricular pressure causes a pressure gradient between the ventricle and atrium that causes the mitral valve to close. This is quickly followed by closure of the tricuspid valve. This first heart sound may normally split and is related to closure of these two valves. The aortic valve opens as soon as LV pressure rises above the pressure in the aorta. Near the end of systole, the T wave is inscribed and the ventricular muscle starts to relax. The aortic valve closes when the pressure in the left ventricle falls below the aortic pressure and S2 is produced. The atrioventricular (AV) valves open when pressure inside the relaxing ventricles fall below atrial pressure. A new cycle then begins.

13. **(E)** The kidneys ascend from the pelvis through the arterial fork formed by the umbilical arteries. Occasionally, one of the kidneys fails to pass through the arterial fork and the kidney remains in the pelvis.

14. **(D)** Withdrawal from benzodiazepines and opiates may produce seizures, while the opiate narcotic meperidine (due to conversion to normeperidine) may actually cause seizures in a toxic state. N-hexane may produce a peripheral neuropathy with chronic use.

15. **(D)** A pancreatic pseudocyst is a collection of pancreatic juice and tissue encased by reactive granulation tissue, occurring in or around the pancreas as a consequence of inflammatory pancreatitis. As the name implies, it is not a true cyst. Generally, a single pseudocyst is present, but in more severe cases they may be multiple or large and can be located either within the pancreas or extend into the intra-abdominal space. Pseudocysts generally communicate with the pancreatic duct and therefore can persist for a long time. The majority of pseudocysts develop following acute pancreatitis. Progression may occur, leading to necrosis or an abscess collection. The diagnosis is established radiologically by ultrasonography or CT.

16. **(A)** The patient is likely taking either a beta blocker or a calcium channel blocker. Both are effective treatments for hypertension but can cause slowing of AV node conduction. In this instance, a first-degree AV block is seen and the QRS complex is normal. This is a benign finding and no action need be taken.

17. **(B)** Nicardipine is a dihydropyridine calcium channel blocker. It has minimal effect on the AV node and would not be used in treatment of SVT. Quinidine would rarely be a first-line treatment for SVT in a young healthy person. It is a class Ia antiarrhythmic. It has anticholinergic effects and thus would not cause AV block. Mexiletine is a class Ib antiarrhythmic, which has little effect on impulse generation or propagation. It would not be used to treat SVT.

18. **(B)** Reduction of maternal mortality in the twentieth century was one of the success stories of modern American public health. The ratio (defined as maternal deaths/live births) was 1/100 in 1900 and had fallen to 7/100,000 in 2000.

19. **(A)** Ectopic ACTH syndrome is characterized by extrapituitary ACTH production, usually by a malignant neoplasm. The ectopic ACTH stimulates cortisol secretion from the adrenal gland. Cortisol inhibits ACTH production by the pituitary gland. Excessive levels of ACTH bind to the melanocyte-stimulating hormone receptor

and can cause hyperpigmentation. In this syndrome, cortisol levels are not inhibited by either low-dose or high-dose dexamethasone suppression.

20. **(B)** It is estimated that more than 70% of malignant mesotheliomas are associated with environmental exposure to asbestos. There are two histologic forms of malignant mesothelioma: fibrous and epithelial. Both have a poor prognosis. Although bronchogenic carcinomas also occur more often in asbestos workers, there is still a stronger association with cigarette smoking.

21. **(B)** SPF refers to ultraviolet B protection. The SPF is calculated by comparing the amount of time required to develop erythema in sunscreen-protected skin divided by the time required to develop erythema in unprotected skin.

22. **(C)** Silbutramine is a serotonin reuptake inhibitor that causes appetite suppression. Orlistat, another obesity medication, binds to intestinal fat. Adrenergic agents such as amphetamines increase energy expenditure and favor lean body mass over fat stores. Leptin is a hormone produced by fat cells that suppresses appetite through hypothalamic regulation. There are currently no medications that specifically increase leptin levels.

23. **(C)** Both folic acid deficiency and vitamin B$_{12}$ deficiency can lead to identical hematologic derangements with macrocytic anemia and hypersegmented neutrophils. However, only vitamin B$_{12}$ deficiency leads to neurologic symptoms. In particular, subacute combined degeneration of the dorsal and lateral spinal columns affect vibration and position senses, leading to a symmetric neuropathy and ataxia. It can progress to paraplegia and even bowel and bladder incontinence. In the central nervous system, memory loss and dementia can occur. As stores of vitamin B$_{12}$ are large, its deficiency usually occurs in strict vegetarians or reflects another underlying process such as pernicious anemia, gastric disease, intestinal disorders (e.g., Crohn's disease, ileal resection, bacterial overgrowth), parasitic infestations, and human immunodeficiency virus (HIV) infection.

24. **(B)** A serum alpha-fetoprotein and abdominal ultrasound have been shown to detect early progression to hepatocellular carcinoma and should be performed in a patient with underlying cirrhosis. Hepatitis A has not been shown to progress to cirrhosis. A patient with antibodies to the hepatitis B surface antigen has either been immunized to hepatitis B or has cleared the antigen and would not be likely to progress to cirrhosis. A patient with a strong drinking history, although at risk for the development of cirrhosis, does not necessarily have cirrhosis without biopsy evidence.

25. **(D)** The presentation given is classic for an ectopic pregnancy; however, up to 50% may not have any symptoms prior to tubal rupture. Therefore, an awareness of risk factors is important and should be weighed when deciding to pursue further diagnostic testing such as with transvaginal ultrasound. Highest risks are conferred by a prior history of ectopic pregnancy or the presence of any tubal pathology. Prior tubal surgery and in utero exposure to DES are also considered high-risk factors. Other risk factors include multiple sexual partners, early age of first intercourse, vaginal douching (associated with more infections), history of sexually transmitted diseases (including pelvic inflammatory disease), smoking (more susceptible to infections), and infertility (possible tubal pathology). Contraceptives generally do not increase the risk of an ectopic pregnancy as they reduce the chance of pregnancy, but women who become pregnant while using intrauterine contraceptive devices do have some increased risk.

26. **(C)** Chlorpromazine and other members of this group of medications have been associated with the development of cholestasis. The other medications listed have not been shown to result in the development of cholestasis.

27. **(B)** Colic peaks from ages 1½ to 2 months and by 3 months is less or resolved. About 10% of infants have colic.

28. **(A)** *S. aureus* is the most commonly isolated organism in osteomyelitis in all age groups. *E. coli* is frequently isolated in infants, *H. influenzae* and *S. pyogenes* are frequently cultured in children over age 1, and *M. tuberculosis* is usually isolated in immunosuppressed patients.

29. **(A)** The most common causes of AVN of the femoral head and humeral head are corticosteroid use, alcohol, and sickle cell anemia. AVN of the lunate and medial femoral condyle is idiopathic in terms of cause.

30. **(B)** The most common malignant germ cell tumor in the mediastinum is the seminoma. It arises purportedly from germ cells that do not migrate normally during embryonic development. A seminoma arising in the mediastinum is identical to a seminoma in the testes.

31. **(E)** The causative agent of oral hairy leukoplakia is Epstein-Barr virus. It occurs almost exclusively in patients with acquired immune deficiency syndrome (AIDS).

32. **(C)** In achalasia there is a reduced or absent motility pattern in the lower two thirds of the esophagus and frequently an elevated LES pressure.

33. **(D)** Infiltrating ductal carcinoma is the most common form of breast cancer, accounting for approximately 70% of breast cancers. Intraductal (in situ) carcinoma and medullary carcinoma are about 10%. Papillary and mucinous carcinomas are less than 3%.

34. **(B)** The L3 root provides sensation to the upper anterior thigh and medial knee and innervates part of the knee extensors. The L4 root provides sensation to most of the anterior thigh, knee, and down the lower leg to the medial ankle. It innervates most of the knee extensors and is primarily responsible for the knee jerk reflex. The L5 root provides sensation to the lateral calf and dorsal and plantar aspects of the foot. It innervates the ankle dorsiflexors and is best checked by testing extensor hallucis longus strength. The S1 root provides sensation to the posterior thigh, lower leg, and lateral ankle. It innervates the ankle plantar flexors and is responsible for the ankle jerk reflex. The S2 root provides sensation to part of the perianal area and provides part of the innervation of the urinary bladder.

35. **(E)** A good history and physical exam can determine the etiology of syncope in most patients. This includes obtaining information about drug and alcohol use and potential familial history of arrhythmias or sudden death. An ECG quickly screens for obvious abnormalities such as Wolff-Parkinson-White syndrome, heart block, prolonged QT syndrome, or prior MI. As a screening tool, the CT scan of the head is very low yield and expensive.

36–37. **(36-B, 37-A)** While conduction can proceed via diffusion through the axon, this is much slower than saltatory conduction in which the charge "jumps" between the exposed axon between segments of myelin. At the node of Ranvier, there is a higher proportion of sodium channels, while potassium channels are more numerous at the myelinated segment of axon. Myelinated nerve fibers conduct much faster than nonmyelinated fibers such as the C-fibers, which carry pain input. Demyelinating neuropathies, such as Guillain-Barré syndrome, are manifest as slowed nerve conductions and often produce a cessation of impulse transmission along the axon, the so-called conduction block.

38. **(C)** The parafollicular C cells are neuroendocrine cells derived from the fourth pharyngeal pouch and the ultimobranchial body. They fuse with the thyroid gland, which is derived from an endodermal thickening in the floor of the primitive pharynx. Follicular cells do not produce calcitonin, and C cells

do not produce thyroglobulin. Both reach the basement membrane of the thyroid follicle; C cells are not exposed to the follicular lumen. TSH regulates follicular cells, but calcium levels regulate calcitonin secretion from C cells.

39. **(A)** Patients with functional bowel disease may have diarrhea, constipation, bloating, and, on occasion, diarrhea alternating with constipation. A typical alarm symptom would be weight loss.

40. **(D)** Figure 7.5 shows red cell fragments and polychromasia consistent with a hemolytic anemia. Hemolytic–uremic syndrome with fragmentation hemolysis and thrombocytopenia can occur after the administration of chemotherapy, and mitomycin is known to do this weeks to months after therapy. Renal involvement is always present and associated with hypertension. Treatment is plasmapheresis.

41. **(D)** The thyroid is connected to the tongue for a short time by the thyroglossal duct. The thyroglossal duct has normally degenerated and disappeared by 7 weeks. Its opening at the base of the tongue is called the *foramen cecum*. The thyroid gland is derived from an endodermal thickening in the floor of the primitive pharynx and is the first endocrine gland to appear in development.

42. **(A)** All the other statements are correct. CABG has been shown to relieve angina above that which is seen with medical therapy.

43. **(A)** Human herpesvirus type 8 has been implicated in the pathogenesis of Kaposi's sarcoma.

44. **(A)** Psychogenic polydipsia is unlikely as the patient is unresponsive and also because the serum osmolality is abnormally elevated. SIADH causes hyponatremia and would increase the urine osmolality. DM is usually evident from glucose levels. The clinical scenario is best compatible with DI, which is a state in which antidiuretic hormone (ADH) activity is absent, either from its absolute deficiency (central) or from resistance to its action (nephrogenic). Before DI is entertained, a water restriction test should generally be performed. This will act to increase the serum osmolality and maximally stimulate ADH release. Consequently, the urine osmolality should also increase as the ADH acts to conserve free water and normalize the serum osmolality. In DI, the urine osmolality will be abnormally low despite an increase in serum osmolality. In central DI, administration of exogenous ADH in the form of DDAVP or vasopressin will act to appropriately increase the urine osmolality but will have little or no effect in patients with nephrogenic DI.

45. **(B)** The only intervention to improve mortality with respect to mechanical ventilation in patients with ARDS is a low-tidal-volume strategy. Improvement of oxygenation by any modality has not been shown to improve mortality, and at FiO_2 greater than 60%, the oxygen may be toxic to the lungs. ARDS is a heterogeneous process mostly affecting the dependent areas of the lung. By proning the patient, perfusion could be delivered to less affected areas of the lung, improving the ventilation–perfusion (V/Q) mismatch. Nitric oxide can also improve V/Q mismatch by preferentially providing vasodilation to areas that are better ventilated. Increasing PEEP acts to recruit more alveoli to aid in gas exchange.

46. **(B)** BNP secreted from the ventricles of the heart rises in response to ventricular stress in terms of increased filling pressures and/or volumes. Although identified as a potential important diagnostic and therapeutic tool in patients with CHF, it can be increased by any condition in which the ventricles are stressed. For example, advanced chronic obstructive pulmonary disease (COPD) with a component of cor pulmonale may lead to elevations in the BNP, as can right ventricular strain from an acute pulmonary embolism.

47. **(A)** Infectious complications occur generally in the earlier post-transplant period. Insidious dyspnea with declining spirometry is suggestive of BO or CB in a patient who has undergone transplantation. Thought to represent a form of chronic rejection, the small airways become partially or completely occluded by fibromyxoid granulation tissue. The mosaic pattern seen on CT represents this patchy small airway disease leading to regional air trapping. This can be more readily identified by obtaining inspiratory and expiratory views. CMV has been loosely associated with the development of BO. Treatment options are limited, so careful management of immunosuppression and aggressive management of episodes of rejection as a means of preventing the development of CB is essential. BOOP or COP tends to be an alveolar process and causes more frequently a restrictive defect on pulmonary function tests.

48. **(C)** The pulmonary arteries provides for the vascular bed supplying the alveoli where gas exchange occurs. However, the systemic blood supply to the lungs originating from the aorta or the intercostal arteries is provided for by the bronchial circulation. These arteries travel adjacent to the bronchi and bronchioles and therefore account for most causes of hemoptysis associated with airway diseases such as bronchiectasis. If localization of the source is possible, embolization therapy is effective in controlling the hemoptysis.

49. **(E)** Chromosome 19 is affected in myotonic dystrophy. In the diseases manifest as trinucleotide repeats (also including Fragile X syndrome and Huntington's disease), the number of repeats of a triplet pattern of nucleic acids correlates with disease severity. With each succeeding generation, the number of repeats and therefore disease severity increases. This is called *anticipation.*

50. **(D)** The clinical features are compatible with mitochondrial disorder. With intact glycolysis, the patient would have no difficulties with anaerobic exercise but would develop symptoms with aerobic exercise. Short stature, retinitis pigmentosa, hearing loss, cerebellar ataxia, and cardiac conduction delay are some of the associated clinical signs and symptoms. The majority of mitochondrial disorders follow maternal inheritance, as children receive all of their mitochondria from the mother.

Practice Test 8
Questions

DIRECTIONS (Questions 1 through 50): Each of the numbered items or incomplete statements in this section is followed by answers or by completions of the statement. Select the ONE answer or completion that is BEST in each case.

1. A 50-year-old woman with a past history of chronic reflux esophagitis presents to her primary care physician with a chief complaint of hoarseness. She admits to awakening from sleep with refluxed gastric juice. Indirect laryngoscopy performed in the office reveals erythema involving the posterior larynx and arytenoids. A presumptive diagnosis of reflux laryngitis is made. The most appropriate treatment for this condition is

    (A) total laryngectomy
    (B) Nissen fundoplication
    (C) barium esophagram
    (D) empiric treatment with high-dose proton pump inhibitors (PPIs) for 3 months
    (E) Mylanta and dietary restrictions

2. A 35-year-old white man has a history of myocardial infarction (MI). His brother and father also had heart attacks in their 30s. The patient has tendinous xanthomas on physical exam. His low-density lipoprotein (LDL) cholesterol is 350 mg/dL. His triglycerides and high-density lipoprotein (HDL) are within normal limits. Which of the following is the most likely genetic abnormality present in this patient?

    (A) deficiency of lipoprotein lipase
    (B) defect in the apo E apolipoprotein
    (C) deficiency of LDL receptors
    (D) absence of apo B apolipoprotein
    (E) excess of LDL receptors

3. Myotoma congenita and ciguatera toxicity are disorders caused by dysfunction of a channel. Which of the following is another disorder with the same cause?

    (A) amyotrophic lateral sclerosis (ALS)
    (B) tardive dyskinesia
    (C) hyperkalemic periodic paralysis
    (D) gout
    (E) migraine

4. A patient may safely take oral contraceptives (OCs) with which of the following conditions?

    (A) active thromboembolic disease
    (B) uncontrolled hypertension
    (C) asthma
    (D) recently diagnosed breast cancer
    (E) endometrial cancer

5. A cystic mass is present on the dorsum of the wrist of a 28-year-old woman. The most likely diagnosis is

    (A) schwannoma
    (B) ganglion
    (C) leiomyosarcoma
    (D) giant cell tumor of tendon sheath origin
    (E) mesothelioma

6. A diagnosis of achalasia can be made using which of the following manometric criteria?

   (A) aperistalsis of the body of the esophagus
   (B) high-amplitude contractions of the body of the esophagus
   (C) a low resting upper esophageal sphincter (UES) pressure
   (D) a high resting UES pressure
   (E) rapid high-amplitude smooth muscle contractions

7. You decide to treat a patient with extensive Paget's. What would the best treatment be?

   (A) estrogens
   (B) raloxifene
   (C) alendronate
   (D) teriparatide
   (E) calcium

8. The most important prognostic factor for human cancer is

   (A) stage
   (B) mitotic index
   (C) vascular invasion
   (D) lymphocytic infiltration
   (E) grade

9. An anterior dislocation of the shoulder is most likely to injure which of the following nerves?

   (A) median
   (B) axillary
   (C) musculocutaneous
   (D) radial
   (E) ulnar

10. Which of the following is associated directly with fracture nonunion?

   (A) nonsteroidial anti-inflammatory use
   (B) tobacco use
   (C) alcohol consumption
   (D) low calcium intake
   (E) low vitamin B_{12} level

11. A 35-year-old woman has a body mass index (BMI) of 28 kg/m^2. She is

   (A) underweight
   (B) normal
   (C) overweight
   (D) obese
   (E) morbidly obese

12. An obese patient wants to take orlistat for weight loss. What is the mechanism of action of this drug?

   (A) serotonin reuptake inhibitor
   (B) lipase inhibitor
   (C) norepinephrine antagonist
   (D) leptin antagonist
   (E) binding to fat molecules

13. Which of the following is associated with an increase in fracture union?

   (A) increased vitamin D intake
   (B) increased calcium intake
   (C) electric field
   (D) high protein diet
   (E) increased vitamin B_{12} intake

14. During exercise in a normal 22-year-old woman, which of the following physiologic changes occurs?

   (A) Arterial pulse pressure is increased.
   (B) Arterial pulse pressure is decreased.
   (C) Arterial pulse pressure is unchanged.
   (D) Arterial pulse is absent.
   (E) Arterial pulse increases and decreases.

15. Which of the following factors could contribute to improved compliance in a patient with diabetes?

   (A) large number of medications
   (B) frequent medication dosing
   (C) high cost of prescriptions
   (D) depression
   (E) attending diabetic teaching classes

16. Cold pain is carried by which nerve fiber type?

   (A) A-alpha
   (B) A-beta
   (C) A-delta

(D) B

(E) C

17. At age 30 your patient's blood pressure was 120/76. At age 70, his pressure is 136/70. This has occurred because of which of the following?

(A) development of hypertension

(B) development of aortic insufficiency

(C) decrease in stroke volume

(D) decrease in arterial compliance

(E) development of diastolic dysfunction

18. Which of the following cholesterol abnormalities would be expected in a patient with low apolipoprotein CII levels?

(A) low LDL

(B) low triglycerides

(C) high LDL

(D) low HDL

(E) high triglycerides

19. A 55-year-old woman is receiving doxorubicin for treatment of malignant lymphoma. She has received several doses of the drug and comes to the office complaining of chest pain and shortness of breath 3 days after her last dose. Regarding her management at this time, which of the following is correct?

(A) A diagnosis of myocardial ischemia is extremely unlikely.

(B) She has a greater than 50% chance of having a drug-induced cardiomyopathy.

(C) Drug-induced cardiomyopathy with doxorubicin does not occur unless > 500 mg/m^2 is given.

(D) Nitrates are used to prevent the cardiotoxicity of doxorubicin.

(E) Doxorubicin can lead to myocardial oxidative stress secondary to free radical formation.

20. The cytologic abnormalities of malignant cells can be explained by

(A) excessive mucin content

(B) cell surface alterations

(C) mitotic activity

(D) chromosomal anomalies

(E) hypercellular DNA (deoxyribonucleic acid) alterations

21. Which of the following systemic therapies used in dermatology requires intermittent liver biopsies to monitor for hepatotoxicity?

(A) cyclosporine

(B) methotrexate

(C) acitretin

(D) tacrolimus

(E) thalidomide

Questions 22 and 23

Refer to Figure 8.1 for questions 22 and 23.

22. A 47-year-old man has had increasing dyspnea. He has a 50-pack-year smoking history, and his family history is strong for premature emphysema. A chest radiograph is performed and reveals hyperinflation. An alpha$_1$-antitrypsin level is obtained and found to be abnormally low. In Figure 8.1, a pulmonary function test is likely to show which type of flow-volume curve?

(A) A

(B) B

(C) C

(D) both A and B

(E) B with a lower peak

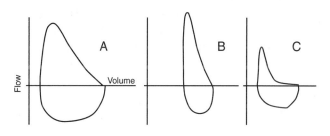

Figure 8.1

23. A 57-year-old woman has had increasing dyspnea on exertion over the past 3 years. She denies any prior smoking. Examination reveals crackles diffusely but most prominent at the bases. Clubbing is noted. There is no sign of congestive heart failure (CHF) otherwise. A chest x-ray reveals diffuse interstitial infiltrates that are mostly basilar and peripheral. A high-resolution computed tomographic (CT) scan confirms a diffuse fibrotic process that is again mostly peripheral and basilar with subpleural honeycombing. From Figure 8.1, what is the likely shape of the flow-volume curve for this patient?

   (A) A
   (B) B
   (C) C
   (D) A (with nasal oxygen given at 2 L/min)
   (E) A (with nasal oxygen given at 4 L/min)

24. Which of the following studies would not provide useful information in establishing a diagnosis of gastroesophageal reflux disease (GERD)?

   (A) upper endoscopy
   (B) 24-hour pH monitoring
   (C) CT of the chest and abdomen
   (D) empiric trial with a PPI
   (E) alteration of diet

25. A 55-year-old woman has dyspnea on exertion. She denies any prior smoking history or occupational exposures. A chest x-ray and an electrocardiogram (ECG) are normal. Because of persistent symptoms, extensive testing had been performed, including echocardiograms, cardiac stress tests, high-resolution CT of the chest, and a ventilation–perfusion (V/Q) scan, all of which were normal. She is severely obese and mildly kyphotic. She denies any regular exercise program. The patient is suspected to have deconditioning as the cause of her dyspnea. However, her pulmonary function test reveals a mild restrictive ventilatory pattern with a reduction in the patient's total lung capacity. What is the likely cause of this finding?

   (A) deconditioning
   (B) idiopathic pulmonary fibrosis

   (C) CHF
   (D) thoracic kyphosis and obesity
   (E) COPD from smoking

26. Which of the following would be regarded as the least complete method to perform colorectal cancer screening in an appropriate patient?

   (A) testing stools for occult blood on three separate occasions
   (B) colonoscopy
   (C) flexible sigmoidoscopy
   (D) physical examination
   (E) barium enema

27. A 65-year-old previously healthy man undergoes a colonoscopic examination and a 4-cm sessile polyp is identified and removed with cauterization in the descending colon. Pathology of the lesion shows the polyp to be a tubulovillous adenoma with low-grade dysplasia. Which of the following would be appropriate for the management of this patient?

   (A) repeat colonoscopy in 3 months
   (B) hemicolectomy
   (C) repeat colonoscopy in 2 weeks
   (D) repeat colonoscopy in 5 years
   (E) yearly colonoscopy for 5 years

28. Patients with ulcerative colitis involving the entire colon (i.e., pancolitis) for more than 20 years are predisposed to

   (A) colon cancer
   (B) gastroesophageal reflux disease (GERD)
   (C) cholecystitis
   (D) Crohn's disease
   (E) colonic rupture

29. A 73-year-old man is admitted to the hospital because of a routine bloodwork showing a sodium of 120 mEq/L. He is fully alert and oriented and otherwise denies any symptoms. His examination reveals that he is clinically euvolemic. A chest x-ray reveals a right superior hilar mass with atelecatasis of the right upper lobe. A diagnosis of small cell lung cancer is made based on a bronchoscopic needle biopsy

of an enlarged subcarinal lymph node. What is the patient's urine osmolality likely to be?

(A) 100 mOsm/L
(B) 600 mOsm/L
(C) 200 mOsm/L
(D) 50 mOsm/L
(E) under 25 mOsm/L

Questions 30 and 31

A 65-year-old man presents to your office with a chief complaint of hoarseness. He also describes waking up frequently at night with water brash and regurgitation of gastric contents that he senses in this throat. He states that his symptoms improve transiently with antacids. The patient has no history of smoking or alcohol use.

30. Which of the following is the most likely diagnosis?

(A) laryngeal cancer
(B) pulmonary asthma
(C) peptic ulcer disease
(D) GERD with associated laryngitis
(E) vocal cord polyp

31. What would be the most appropriate course of therapy?

(A) referral for laryngectomy
(B) empiric therapy with a PPI
(C) increasing the dosage and frequency of the antacid therapy
(D) barium swallow
(E) polyp removal

32. A 45-year-old woman with obstructive hypertrophic cardiomyopathy has an episode of atrial fibrillation. Which of the following treatments is contraindicated?

(A) cardioversion
(B) lidocaine
(C) amiodarone
(D) digoxin
(E) verapamil

33. Which skin layer contains the majority of melanocytes?

(A) stratum basalis
(B) stratum corneum
(C) stratum granulosum
(D) stratum spinulosum
(E) stratum superior

34. Regarding pacemakers in patients with conduction system disease, which of the following is correct?

(A) Pacemakers function by recognizing native electrical activity of the heart and suppressing it.
(B) A single-chamber atrial pacemaker is appropriate for a patient with atrial fibrillation and symptomatic bradycardia.
(C) Pacemakers are indicated only when the level of heart block is felt to be in the distal conduction system.
(D) Pacemakers are useful in terminating potentially lethal arrhythmias.
(E) A single-chamber atrial pacemaker is appropriate in a patient with sick sinus syndrome only.

35. Which of the following is the most common tumor in bone?

(A) osteogenic sarcoma
(B) multiple myeloma
(C) Ewing's sarcoma
(D) osteoid osteoma
(E) metastatic tumors

36. What is the description of the pattern of pulmonary function tests (PFTs) in a patient with asthma or chronic obstructive pulmonary disease (COPD)?

(A) restrictive—parenchymal
(B) restrictive—extraparenchymal
(C) normal
(D) obstructive
(E) restrictive only

37. A 60-year-old woman is admitted with swollen legs. Her lung fields are clear to auscultation, but her neck veins are elevated and her liver is somewhat enlarged. A systolic murmur is heard, which increases during inspiration. Her diagnosis is

   (A) mitral regurgitation
   (B) mitral stenosis and biventricular failure
   (C) systolic failure
   (D) left heart failure
   (E) right heart failure

38. A 20-year-old man with a history of type 1 diabetes stopped taking his insulin while he was on vacation. He developed abdominal pain, nausea, and vomiting and was found to have a glucose of 500 and a metabolic acidosis. Which of the following statements is true regarding diabetic ketoacidosis?

   (A) Ketone bodies are not derived from excess free fatty acids.
   (B) Acetone is used by the body as fuel.
   (C) Excess ketone bodies lead to a high anion gap metabolic alkalosis.
   (D) Ketone bodies cannot be used by the brain as fuel.
   (E) Hepatic hydroxymethylglutaryl coenzyme A (HMG-CoA) synthase is the rate-limiting step in the synthesis of ketone bodies.

39. Regarding cardiac manifestations of systemic lupus erythematosus (SLE), which of the following is correct?

   (A) Cardiac manifestations are more common clinically than at autopsy.
   (B) The most common cardiac manifestation of lupus is pericarditis, which is seen in up to 30% of patients with active disease.
   (C) Myocarditis is clinically present in over 50% of patients with lupus.
   (D) Epicardial lesions called Libman-Sacks lesions affect the epicardium in 90% of lupus patients.
   (E) Septal rupture is common.

40. Which of the following etiologic associations with human acute leukemia has been proven?

   (A) irradiation
   (B) uncooked seafood
   (C) red meat
   (D) viruses
   (E) estrogen

41. Which skin layer contains cells lacking nuclei?

   (A) stratum basalis
   (B) stratum corneum
   (C) stratum granulosum
   (D) stratum spinulosum
   (E) all layers have nuclei

42. A 34-year-old previously healthy woman develops progressive dyspnea. Her chest x-ray was read as normal. An echocardiogram, however, identifies severe pulmonary hypertension. No cause for the pulmonary hypertension is found, and she is diagnosed with primary pulmonary hypertension. If a PFT were performed, what would be the appearance of the flow-volume curve shown in Figure 8.2?

   (A) A
   (B) B
   (C) C
   (D) B (after beta-agonist therapy)
   (E) B (with oxygen at 2 L/min)

43. Which of the following medications has been associated with the development of pseudomembranous colitis?

   (A) acetaminophen
   (B) naproxen
   (C) azulfidine
   (D) ciprofloxacin
   (E) phenobarbital

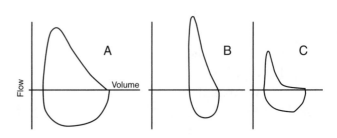

Figure 8.2

44. A 32-year-old man is being followed for peri-anal Crohn's disease. The patient does not have evidence of systemic or colonic disease. Which of the following is the most appropriate treatment for a flare leading to the development of a perianal fistula in this patient?

    (A) conservative treatment with sitz baths
    (B) metronidazole
    (C) erythromycin
    (D) fistulotomy
    (E) penicillin

45. A 40-year-old man falls from an 8-foot ladder, landing on his left foot. By x-ray he has a comminuted os calcis fracture. What other anatomic area is commonly injured in such accidents?

    (A) cervical spine
    (B) dorsal spine
    (C) lumbar spine
    (D) sacrum
    (E) pelvis

46. A 60-year-old woman is mechanically ventilated (volume controlled) for respiratory failure due to severe community-acquired pneumonia. During rounds, the attending points out elevated peak airway pressures. He further places an end-inspiratory pause and determines that the plateau pressure is unchanged. Which of the following could account for the elevated peak airway pressures in this patient?

    (A) mucous plugging and bronchospasm
    (B) elevated blood pressure
    (C) lower inspiratory flows
    (D) noncompliant lungs
    (E) hypotension

47. A patient is admitted to the intensive care unit (ICU) with a documented duodenal ulcer bleed. Which of the following would be useful to know with reference to prognosis of the patient?

    (A) appearance of the ulcer (i.e., clean based versus presence of a visible vessel)
    (B) presence of *Helicobacter pylori*

    (C) the weight of the patient
    (D) the size of the ulcer
    (E) results of blood cultures

48. A 55-year-old man presents to your office with a prior history of *H. pylori* infection leading to peptic ulcer disease. The patient undergoes triple antibiotic therapy and the ulcer heals. Two years later the patient presents again to your office with epigastric pain suggestive of peptic ulcer disease and an endoscopy is performed, which confirms the presence of *H. pylori* by biopsy and an active duodenal ulcer. The correct course of action to treat this patient would include which of the following?

    (A) prohibiting coffee
    (B) re-treating with the same antibiotic regimen
    (C) ordering a urea breath test to confirm the diagnosis of *H. pylori*
    (D) re-treating with a different antibiotic regimen
    (E) using Mylanta four times a day

49. Which of the following statements concerning mutations is correct?

    (A) Insertion of base pairs will not cause mutations.
    (B) Deletions of base pairs may cause mutations.
    (C) Most mutations are caused by thymine dimers.
    (D) Substitutions of base pairs will never cause mutations.
    (E) Transition or transversion is not a cause of mutations.

50. Which of the following pathologic changes would be an unexpected finding on examination of the brain of a patient with dementia of the Alzheimer's type?

    (A) senile plaques
    (B) neurofibrillary tangles
    (C) arteriosclerotic changes
    (D) neuronal loss
    (E) amyloid deposition

Answers and Explanations

1. **(D)** This case represents extraesophageal manifestations of GERD. Endoscopically, there is posterior commissural erythema as well as erythema of the arytenoids. The treatment of choice for reflux laryngitis includes high-dose PPI therapy for at least 3 months. The other choices listed would not be definitive therapy for reflux laryngitis.

2. **(C)** Familial hypercholesterolemia, the most likely diagnosis in this patient, is due to a deficiency in LDL receptors on cell membranes and a resulting inability to clear LDL cholesterol from the circulation. A deficiency of lipoprotein lipase leads to elevated chylomicrons. Patients with abnormalities in apo E levels (familial dysbetalipoproteinemia) have elevated remnants of very-low-density lipoprotein (VLDL) and chylomicrons. Absence of apo B leads to absence of chylomicrons, VLDL, and LDL.

3. **(E)** Myotonia congenita, a chloride channelopathy, is an autosomal recessive or dominant disorder characterized by clinical myotonia (slow relaxation of muscle), absence of muscle weakness, and cramping pains worse with cold exposure. Ciguatera is a toxin that blocks sodium channels.

4. **(C)** While theophylline levels can be affected by OC administration, this does not mean that patients with asthma can't use this method as long as their levels are closely monitored. Endometrial and breast cancers are often estrogen dependent and therefore OCs, which contain estrogen, and progesterone are contraindicated with these conditions. Both hypertension and deep venous thrombosis are potential complications of OC use, and, therefore, when these conditions are already present, their use is contraindicated.

5. **(B)** A ganglion is the only mass listed that is cystic. Ganglion cysts occur most commonly on the dorsum of the wrist and will transilluminate with a penlight.

6. **(A)** In most cases of achalasia, although the clinical and radiographic findings may suggest the diagnosis of achalasia, it is imperative to obtain a manometric examination. There are three major manometric features of achalasia:

    1. Elevated resting lower esophageal sphincter (LES) pressure (generally > 45 mmHg).

    2. Incomplete LES relaxation. In the normal esophagus there is generally complete relaxation of the LES following swallowing. However, in achalasia there is incomplete or absent relaxation of the LES.

    3. Aperistalsis occurs when the smooth muscle portion of the body of the esophagus fails to contract normally in response to swallowing. In the majority of patients the contractions are of low amplitude.

7. **(C)** Bisphosphonates are the treatment of choice for Paget's disease.

8. **(A)** The stage of the disease is the most important prognostic factor. Stage refers to the extent of disease in the patient and includes local, regional, or distant spread. Tumor grade

or differentiation, mitotic count, and extent of vascular invasion correlate with stage of the tumor and contribute to prognosis.

9. **(B)** Any of the nerves listed can be injured during a shoulder dislocation. The axillary nerve courses from the quadrangular space in the posterior shoulder around the lateral and anterior aspect of the proximal humerus, rendering it prone to injury during anterior dislocation. A throrough neurologic exam should be performed prior to joint reduction.

10. **(B)** Tobacco use in any form is strongly associated with delayed union and nonunion of fractures secondary to the vascular effects of nicotine. Excessive alcohol consumption and low calcium intake may reflect a general malnutrition, which can affect fracture union. These factors alone generally do not affect union.

11. **(C)** BMI of 20 to 26 is desirable for adults; 27–29 is moderately overweight; 30–40 is obese; and over 40 is morbidly obese.

12. **(B)** Orlistat inhibits absorption of fat through its inhibitory effect on pancreatic lipase.

13. **(C)** Bone has an inherent electrical field in the milliamp range. Bending a long bone increases that current. Bone growth stimulators (implantable and external) are commonly used to treat nonunions.

14. **(A)** Pulse pressure equals systolic blood pressure minus diastolic blood pressure. Pulse pressure is determined by the elasticity of the arteries and stroke volume. Elasticity is unchanged by exercise, but stroke volume increases. Therefore, pulse pressure increases.

15. **(E)** Patients with diabetes may have trouble adhering to a given treatment regimen for many reasons, including having a long medication list and having to take a medication more than one or two times a day. If a patient is not experiencing symptoms related to the diabetes, it may be difficult to adhere to a strict medication regimen. Depression may

also contribute to noncompliance and occurs with increased frequency in patients with diabetes.

16. **(C)** Both warm pain and pinprick are carried by the nonmyelinated, slow-conducting C-fiber, while the large, myelinated A-alpha fiber carries proprioception and vibration sensation.

17. **(D)** With aging, the compliance of major arteries decreases. With stiffening, the pulse pressure increases. (Pulse pressure equals systolic blood pressure minus diastolic blood pressure). There is a slight increase in the systolic pressure owing to injection of blood into less compliant vessels. The diastolic pressure is slightly lowered as blood is rapidly transmitted out of the large vessels resulting in lowered blood volume at the end of diastole. Additional vascular changes seen in the elderly include arteriolar vasoconstrictions, an increase in total peripheral resistance, and an increase in mean arterial pressure.

18. **(E)** Apolipoprotein CII serves as a cofactor to lipoprotein lipase (LPL). LPL is located on the capillary endothelium and removes triglycerides from chylomicrons for storage and utilization. Deficiency of either LPL or CII leads to decreased clearance and elevated plasma levels of triglycerides.

19. **(E)** Doxorubicin cardiomyopathy is generally dose related. While rare at lower doses, it is seen in 30 to 40% of patients receiving ≥ 700 mg/m^2. Drug-induced ischemia and infarction have been associated with mg/m^2. The cardiomyopathy of doxorubicin is felt to be related to oxidative stress secondary to increased free radical formation.

20. **(D)** Alterations in the nucleus that reflect chromosomal changes such as increased size and abnormal shape are diagnostic of malignancies. Although cell surface alterations can give rise to cytologic abnormalities, they are not diagnostic. Mitotic figures are not specific for cancer. The presence of mucin does not add to whether the tumor is malignant.

21. **(B)** The potential for liver toxicity with the use of methotrexate necessitates serial liver biopsies once a certain cumulative dose of drug is achieved.

22. **(C)** The clinical history is that of premature emphysema even with a 50-pack-year smoking history. The family history and the alpha$_1$-antitrypsin level is suggestive of alpha$_1$-antitrypsin deficiency, and phenotyping should be performed to confirm this. Pulmonary function tests are important in identifying various ventilatory abnormalities including airflow obstruction. The flow-volume curve is typically used to identify these abnormalities. The upper portions of the curve represent flows during forced expiration, and the lower curve shows forced inspiration plotted against the volume. Choice C depicts the typical appearance of an obstructive pattern with reduced peak flows, scalloped or scooped expiratory phase, and a reduced forced vital capacity. A reduction in the ratio of the forced expiratory volume in one second (FEV$_1$) to the forced vital capacity (FVC) defines an obstructive limitation, and the FEV$_1$ itself has been used to quantitate the severity of the obstruction.

23. **(B)** The clinical picture suggests the diagnosis of idiopathic pulmonary fibrosis. This disease can be insidious but is relentless. It falls in the category of disorders termed *interstitial lung diseases* and causes a restrictive ventilatory pattern on pulmonary function testing. The hallmark of restrictive lung disease on pulmonary function testing is a reduction in the total lung capacity, which is also reflected in a symmetric reduction in the FEV$_1$ and FVC. With parenchymal destruction, as occurs in emphysema or pulmonary fibrosis, there is also a reduction in the diffusing capacity. The flow-volume curve of a patient with pulmonary fibrosis should reflect a reduced lung capacity (reduction in the FVC). Therefore, choice B with a narrowing (reflecting smaller volumes) reflects the best answer. Note that the peak flow is preserved given the decreased compliance of the lung ("stiffer" lungs) and the lack of "scooping" as might be seen with a more obstructive pattern.

24. **(C)** An upper endoscopy may disclose esophagitis and the presence of Barrett's esophagus. The most sensitive modality for confirming the presence of GERD is 24-hour monitoring with a pH probe. One study showed that empiric therapy with a PPI is valid for establishing a diagnosis of GERD and is perhaps the most cost-effective strategy for making a diagnosis of GERD. A CT examination of the chest and abdomen would not be useful for making a diagnosis of GERD.

25. **(D)** Deconditioning alone will not be evident on a pulmonary function test. However, both obesity and thoracic kyphosis can cause a restrictive pattern. Restrictive ventilatory patterns can arise due to lung parenchymal abnormalities as in idiopathic pulmonary fibrosis, but can also occur as a result of "chest wall" pathology as in neuromuscular weakness, pleural processes, kyphosis, or obesity. Although interstitial lung disease may be radiographically negative in up to 10% on plain chest x-rays, the high-resolution CT excludes this cause of restrictive lung disease. CHF can cause a variety of changes on the PFT but is easily excluded clinically and based on several of the tests that the patient has already had.

26. **(D)** A careful physical examination alone is insufficient to determine whether the patient is at risk for colorectal cancer. The remaining tests would all be regarded as potentially useful methods.

27. **(A)** Given that the polyp was sessile and had a low-grade dysplasia, a repeat colonoscopy is warranted after the initial edema and inflammation from the cauterization subside (i.e., in 3 months). Therefore, a repeat colonoscopy at 2 weeks would be too soon and a repeat colonoscopy in 5 years would be too long after the procedure.

28. **(A)** Patients with a long history of pancolitis are predisposed to the development of colon cancer, and a decision may need to be made with regard to performing a total or subtotal colectomy. Patients with this disor-

der are not at increased risk for the development of either GERD or Crohn's disease.

29. **(B)** The patient described has euvolemic hyponatremia. Assuming that the patient is indeed hypo-osmolar, the patient's clinical picture is best compatible with SIADH (syndrome of inappropriate antidiuretic hormone secretion). In particular, SIADH is a well-known paraneoplastic phenomenon of small cell lung cancer. In this patient who is hyponatremic, the normal physiologic response is to shut off ADH secretion from the pituitary. This would then have the effect of diluting the urine (hypo-osmolar urine relative to the serum osmolality) and consequently increase the serum osmolality back to normal (approximately 280 mOsm/L). Therefore, the urine osmolality in a person with hypo-osmolar hyponatremia would be to dilute the urine to an osmolality less (usually significantly less) than the serum osmolality. In SIADH, there is an inappropriate excess of ADH which acts to concentrate the urine, leading to the inappropriate retention of free water and thus aggravating the hyponatremia.

30. **(D)** This patient has a diagnosis of GERD with associated laryngitis. The main symptom complex of nighttime heartburn and regurgitation predisposes the larynx and hypopharynx to acid-induced injury. Laryngeal cancer would generally be considered if hoarseness was not associated with reflux. Peptic ulcer disease and asthma would not result in the episodes of regurgitation.

31. **(B)** Generally, empiric therapy with a PPI would be started and treatment would ensue for 2 to 3 months. Should no improvement occur, then a referral to an ear, nose, and throat (ENT) specialist could be considered. Antacid therapy generally provides short-term symptom relief but would not be considered a specific therapy. A barium swallow in the majority of patients with GERD is normal and would therefore not be helpful.

32. **(D)** Cardioversion in an appropriately anti-coagulated patient or in an unstable patient is appropriate. Lidocaine would be ineffective but unlikely to cause harm. Amiodarone, either IV or PO, would slow heart rate and facilitate or result in conversion. It must be used with caution in obstructive hypertrophic cardiomyopathy owing to its afterload-reducing effects. Verapamil would slow heart rate and improve diastolic function. Digoxin, which increases the force of contractility and would increase the degree of obstruction, is contraindicated.

33. **(A)** Most of the epidermal melanocytes are contained in the basal layer.

34. **(E)** Pacemakers function by recognizing native cardiac electrical activity. If the unit senses normal activity, its function is inhibited and no paced beat is created. Pacemakers are implanted in patients with symptomatic bradycardia regardless of the level of heart block. A single-chamber atrial pacemaker would be of use in a patient whose only conduction problem is sick sinus syndrome. As the sinus rate slows, the pacemaker would generate an output to maintain a normal rate. In atrial fibrillation, the problem is with ventricular rate, not atrial rate. The atrium cannot be paced in atrial fibrillation, and an atrial pacemaker would do nothing to protect against bradycardia. Pacemakers alone cannot terminate malignant arrhythmias such as ventricular tachycardia.

35. **(E)** Primary bone tumors are rare. They generally occur above the elbow, above the knee, and in the axial skeleton.

36. **(D)** Patients with asthma or COPD show an obstructive pattern on the PFTs, which will have a depressed FEV_1-to-FVC ratio.

37. **(E)** The murmur described is consistent with tricuspid regurgitation. In isolated right heart failure, signs and symptoms of left heart failure are not present. In right heart failure, the heart's ability to pump blood to the left side is reduced and the left ventricular end-diastolic pressure (LVEDP) may be low. The most common cause of right heart failure is left heart failure. However, right

heart failure can occur as a result of right ventricular infarction, pulmonary embolism, or cor pulmonale. Signs and symptoms of right heart failure include elevated central venous pressure leading to neck vein elevation and hepatic congestion, edema of the lower extremities, and ascites in severe cases.

38. **(E)** The ketone bodies acetoacetate and beta-hydroxybutyrate are formed from excess acetyl CoA, which is derived from excess free fatty acids. The third ketone body, acetone, cannot be metabolized or used by the body as fuel. Excess ketone bodies lead to increased circulating hydrogen ions and a high anion gap metabolic acidosis. Ketone bodies are used by the brain as fuel when levels are sufficiently high. HMG-CoA synthase is the rate-limiting step in ketone body synthesis.

39. **(B)** Clinical lesions with lupus are seen far less frequently than are abnormalities detected at autopsy. Myocarditis is seen in up to 10% of lupus patients. Libman-Sacks lesions are a form of endocardial lesions seen in up to 50% of autopsies performed on patients with lupus.

40. **(A)** Certain antibiotics and benzene, which share certain chemical configurations, have been associated with leukemia development. Chemotherapeutic agents have certainly been found to have leukemogenic potential. Radiation therapy has been linked with leukemia development probably due to stem cell damage with chromosomal aberrations. Viruses have been associated with leukemia but not proven in humans.

41. **(B)** The cells of the stratum corneum are anucleate, and thus are technically dead.

42. **(A)** Pulmonary hypertension will not be reflected on the spirometry aspect of the PFT as it is neither a restrictive nor a ventilatory disorder. However, this may be suggested by a complete PFT when the diffusing capacity is noted to be abnormally low in isolation. If the diffusing capacity is low with a total lung capacity that is increased and an obstructive pattern on the spirometry, then emphysema might be suggested. If the total lung capacity is reduced with the low diffusing capacity, then a lung parenchymal problem such as pulmonary fibrosis might be suggested, but the isolated reduction in the diffusing capacity with normal lung volumes and spirometry is strongly suggestive of a vascular-related phenomenon or possibly anemia. Pulmonary hypertension or chronic thromboembolic disease would be important considerations in this category. Therefore, the flow-volume curve—which graphically represents the spirometry and not the lung volumes or diffusing capacity—should be normal.

43. **(D)** Nearly every antibiotic has been associated with the development of pseudomembranous colitis. None of the other agents listed have been implicated in this disorder.

44. **(B)** Metronidazole (Flagyl) is an appropriate initial therapy for the management of perianal disease in a patient with Crohn's disease. Erythromycin has not been shown to be useful, and, although conservative therapy can be used as an adjunct, it should not be the only therapy directed at the perianal involvement. Fistulotomy should be reserved as a last therapy in the conservative management of this disease.

45. **(C)** Although a thorough physical exam is mandatory in a fall from height, fractures of the upper lumbar spine are common in falls in which a fracture of the os calcis occurs.

46. **(A)** Airway pressure in a mechanically ventilated patient has two basic components: dynamic and static pressures. The total airway pressure is the sum of these two pressures. The dynamic component is generated by the flow of air through the airways and is proportional to the resistance and the rate of air flow ($P = R \times F$). The static pressure is proportional to the volume of the lungs and inversely proportional to the compliance of the lungs ($P = V/C$). Therefore, when air flow is zero at end inspiration, for example, the pressure generated reflects entirely the compliance of the lung at a given volume. This

plateau or static pressure is often determined at bedside by causing an inspiratory pause and measuring the airway pressure. Since this is unchanged, the compliance of the lung is unlikely to be changed. However, the peak airway pressures are higher in this patient. For this to occur, the dynamic component has increased, implying either increased flow rates or increased resistance of the airways to air flow—as might occur with bronchospasm or mucous plugging. Therefore, the best answer is A.

47. **(A)** The most critical factor in determining the risk for ulcer rebleeding is the appearance of the ulcer. A clean ulcer base has a low likelihood of rebleeding, whereas the presence of underlying vessels or presence of active bleeding carries an increased risk for further bleeding. Size of the ulcer may dictate the length of time for the ulcer to heal but has no bearing on risk for rebleeding. Age and presence of comorbid diseases would have a significant impact on the overall prognosis of the patient.

48. **(D)** The patient has recurrent *H. pylori*, which suggests the possibility of resistance to the first antibiotic regimen. The correct course of action, therefore, would be to use a different antibiotic regimen. Avoidance of certain foods or coffee has not been shown to influence the course of disease. If a biopsy confirms the presence of the organisms, then a confirmatory test would not be necessary.

49. **(B)** Mutations are caused by changes in the base sequence of DNA. Substitution of one base pair for another is the most common mutation. Transition or transversions may cause mutations. A transition is replacement of one purine by another purine or a pyrimidine for a pyrimidine. Transverions refer to replacement of a purine with a pyrimidine and vice versa. Frame shift mutations (insertions or deletions) are less common than substitutions. The formation of thymine dimers is not common, and in fact repair mechanims usually deal with this.

50. **(C)** Arteriosclerosis is not a common feature of a brain with Alzheimer's disease but is certainly seen in the vascular dementias. The senile plaque is composed of degenerated, enlarged axon endings with surrounding amyloid. Amyloid may also line the walls of cerebral arterioles. Plaques and tangles appear first and are most numerous in the hippocampus of the limbic system but later appear throughout the cerebral cortex.

Practice Test 9
Questions

1. A 23-year-old woman with anorexia nervosa has not eaten in 2 days. Which of the following is converted to acetyl coenzyme A (CoA) (and therefore not to glucose)?

   (A) free fatty acids
   (B) glycerol
   (C) lactate
   (D) amino acids
   (E) leucine

2. Regarding cardiac muscle metabolism, which of the following statements is correct?

   (A) Cardiac muscle metabolism differs from skeletal muscle metabolism in that the heart has greater ability to generate energy anaerobically.
   (B) Cardiac muscle metabolizes fat efficiently.
   (C) The TCA cycle is operative in anaerobic cardiac tissue.
   (D) During exercise, coronary arteriolar resistance increases.
   (E) Cardiac muscle can function without oxygen.

3. A 19-year-old runner is seen for a routine physical exam. He has no complaints. On physical exam his blood pressure is 108/60 and his pulse is 60. His lungs are clear to auscultation and percussion. His left ventricular impulse is not diffuse. His first heart sound splits with expiration. His second heart sound is normal. There is an apical third heart sound. No fourth heart sound or murmur is noted. No edema is present. The most likely diagnosis is

   (A) normal physical exam in a healthy young athlete
   (B) atrial septal defect
   (C) ventricular septal defect
   (D) dilated cardiomyopathy
   (E) obstructive hypertrophic cardiomyopathy (HCM)

4. A 40-year-old woman presents with tremors and palpitations and is diagnosed with Graves' disease. She is prescribed propylthiouracil. Which of the following best describes the mechanism of action of propylthiouracil on thyroid function?

   (A) It inhibits the action of thyroid-stimulating hormone (TSH).
   (B) It inhibits the uptake of iodide by the thyroid cell.
   (C) It interferes with the coupling of tyrosine residues in the thyroglobulin molecule.
   (D) It inhibits the release of thyroid hormone from the thyroid gland.
   (E) It does not affect tyrosine.

5. Most of the mitotic activity in normal epidermis occurs in the

   (A) stratum basalis
   (B) stratum corneum
   (C) stratum granulosum
   (D) stratum spinulosum
   (E) corneal epithelium

6. A 35-year-old man is asplenic from a distant motor vehicle accident. He does not recall having had any immunizations related to this. What would you suggest?

(A) Avoid the meningococcal polysaccharide vaccines.

(B) Avoid the polyvalent *Streptococcus pneumoniae* vaccine.

(C) Give the hepatitis B vaccine series.

(D) Give the *Haemophilus influenzae* type B vaccine.

(E) It is too late for vaccines.

7. Which of the following leukemias is associated with the t9;22 or Philadelphia chromosome?

(A) acute promyelocytic leukemia (APML)

(B) chronic lymphocytic leukemia (CLL)

(C) erythroleukemia

(D) acute myelogenous leukemia (AML)

(E) chronic myelogenous leukemia (CML)

8. Which structure is responsible for binding epidermal squamous cells to one another?

(A) anchoring fibril

(B) basement membrane

(C) desmosome

(D) hemidesmosome

(E) lamina lucida

9. A 30-year-old male falls 6 feet onto his outstretched right hand. He arrives at the emergency department (ED) holding his arm with the elbow flexed. Capillary refill in his fingers is sluggish, and his radial pulse is absent. X-rays show an anterior dislocation of the elbow. What is the next course of action?

(A) Doppler examination of radial and ulnar arteries

(B) arteriogram

(C) closed reduction applying straight distal traction at the wrist

(D) closed reduction applying distal traction pulling through the proximal forearm with one hand and the protruding olecranon with the other hand with the elbow flexed

(E) open reduction of the dislocation

10. Which of the following disease processes is associated with high urine levels of hydroxyproline?

(A) Paget's disease

(B) fibrous dysplasia

(C) multiple myeloma

(D) osteoporosis

(E) ostoegenesis imperfecta

11. During fibrinolysis, which of the following substances splits the fibrin molecule into products of varying molecular size?

(A) plasminogen

(B) plasmin

(C) antiplasmin

(D) proactivator

(E) activator

12. The most common bacterial cause of osteomyelitis is

(A) *Escherichia coli*

(B) *Salmonella typhi*

(C) *Staphylococcus aureus*

(D) *Mycobacterium tuberculosis*

(E) *Proteus mirabilis*

Questions 13 and 14

A 53-year-old man with a history of hypertension is admitted with nausea, vomiting, and epigastric pain. His vital signs on admission are: heart rate 90, BP 90/60, temperature 37.2°C (99°F), and respiratory rate 18. He is cold, clammy, and anxious. His electrocardiogram (ECG) is shown in Figure 9.1.

13. This patient's diagnosis most likely is

(A) acute anterior myocardial infarction (MI)

(B) acute closure of the left anterior descending coronary artery

(C) acute lateral wall MI secondary to closure of the right coronary artery

(D) acute inferior MI with right ventricular involvement

(E) aortic dissection

14. A 43-year-old man presents with easy bruising, muscle weakness, centripetal obesity,

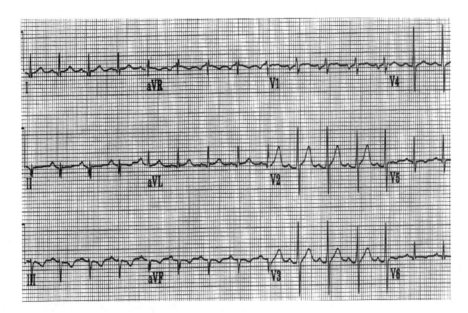

Figure 9.1

and facial plethora. You suspect Cushing's syndrome. A 24-hour urine free cortisol is very high. Plasma adrenocorticotropic hormone (ACTH) is low. What is the next step?

(A) magnetic resonance imaging (MRI) of the pituitary

(B) high-dose dexamethasone suppression test

(C) overnight dexamethasone suppression test

(D) computed tomographic (CT) scan of the adrenals

(E) CT scan of the chest

15. Osteoporosis is associated with which of the following?

(A) Osteoclastic activity continues at a normal rate, and osteoblastic activity is diminished.

(B) Osteoblastic and osteoclastic activity continues at a normal rate.

(C) Osteoclastic activity is diminished, and osteoblastic activity continues at a normal rate.

(D) Osteoclastic activity is increased, and osteoblastic activity continues at a normal rate.

(E) excessive calcium intake

16. A 25-year-old man who is 62″ tall wants to increase his height and requests a prescription for growth hormone. Which of the following effects will growth hormone administration have on this man?

(A) It will increase his height by only 8% to 10%.

(B) It will decrease intestinal calcium absorption.

(C) It will cause low blood sugars.

(D) It will increase insulin-like growth factor-1 (IGF-1) levels.

(E) It will decrease amino acid uptake by skeletal muscle.

17. Which of the above leukemias is associated with 15;17 translocation?

(A) APML

(B) CLL

(C) erythroleukemia

(D) AML

(E) CML

18. A 36-year-old woman becomes pregnant. A serum screen for Down syndrome (trisomy 21) returns abnormal and the diagnosis is confirmed by prenatal cytogenetics testing from an amniocentesis. Which of the following is true of Down syndrome?

(A) Incidence of trisomy 21 decreases with maternal age.
(B) Down syndrome is familial.
(C) There is a decreased incidence of congenital heart disease, such as septal defects.
(D) There is a decreased incidence of acute leukemias.
(E) There is a decreased incidence of Alzheimer's disease.

19. In fracture healing, endochondral ossification refers to

(A) bone formation from cartilage
(B) periosteal new bone formation
(C) bone formation from chondrocytes
(D) bone formation directly from stem cells
(E) bone formation directly on fracture hematoma

20. A 25-year-old woman presents with weight loss, fatigue, amenorrhea, hypoglycemia, and hyponatremia. You suspect adrenal insufficiency. You do a cosyntropin stimulation test: 60 minutes after injecting 250 µg of cosyntropin, you draw a serum cortisol. A normal response is defined as a serum cortisol of at least

(A) 10 µg/dL
(B) 20 µg/dL
(C) 30 µg/dL
(D) 40 µg/dL
(E) 100 µg/dL

21. What is the structure indicated by the arrow in Figure 9.2?

(A) musculocutaneous nerve
(B) ulnar nerve
(C) axillary nerve
(D) radial nerve
(E) median nerve

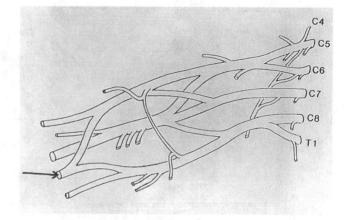

Figure 9.2

22. A patient with suspected adrenal insufficiency fails a cosyntropin stimulation test. What is the next step?

(A) MRI of the pituitary
(B) 24-hour urine free cortisol
(C) ACTH level
(D) CT scan of the adrenals
(E) glucose tolerance test

23. Which structure is responsible for connecting the epidermal keratinocytes to the basement membrane?

(A) anchoring fibril
(B) basement membrane fibrin
(C) desmosome
(D) hemidesmosome
(E) lamina lucida

24. A 70-year-old man presents to you with a history of iron-deficiency anemia but denies blood per rectum or melena. The patient is otherwise healthy and denies taking aspirin or nonsteroidal anti-inflammatory agents (NSAIDs). A stool examination is positive for occult blood. A colonoscopy is performed, which is negative for polyp or malignancy. Which of the following would be the most appropriate course of action?

(A) barium enema
(B) upper endoscopy
(C) bone marrow aspiration
(D) bleeding scan
(E) CT of abdomen

25. Which of the following tests would be most helpful in evaluating chest pain in a 58-year-old man with long-standing hypertension?

    (A) stress ECG
    (B) coronary arteriography
    (C) echocardiogram
    (D) stress echocardiogram
    (E) CT cardiac scan

26. Lyme disease is characterized by which of the following?

    (A) women are affected more than men
    (B) autoimmune disease
    (C) metacarpophalangeal joints are more often affected than interphalangeal joints
    (D) systemic illness is common
    (E) erythema marginatum

27. Wolff's law of bone concerns which of the following?

    (A) Bone becomes electrically charged when subjected to mechanical stress.
    (B) Disuse of bone leads to osteoporosis.
    (C) When stress is applied to bone, trabeculae develop and align themselves to adapt to those lines of stress.
    (D) Distraction at a fracture site lessens the formation of callus and delays union.
    (E) Bone heals with bone and not scar tissue.

28. The 56-year-old woman pictured in Figure 9.3 has hypertension and diabetes. She has gained 50 pounds in the last 6 months without a change in her diet or activity level. A 24-hour urine free cortisol is ordered and found to be markedly elevated. An ACTH level is mildly elevated. The patient is noted to have abdominal striae, osteoporosis on dual-energy x-ray absorptiometry (DEXA) scan, a history of poor wound healing, and muscle weakness. What condition do you suspect?

    (A) hypothyroidism
    (B) renal failure

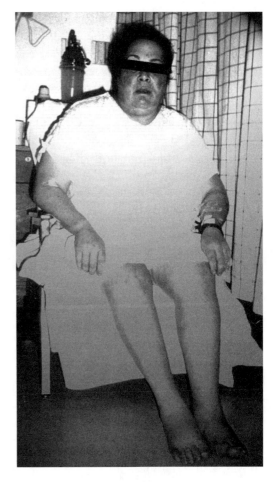

Figure 9.3

    (C) hyperaldosteronism
    (D) pseudo-pseudoparathyroidism
    (E) Cushing's disease

29. Which of the following human insulin preparations has the shortest duration of action?

    (A) insulin Lispro
    (B) regular
    (C) Neutral Protamine Hagedorn (NPH)
    (D) Ultralente
    (E) Humalog

30. A 23-year-old female medical student decides to begin jogging. She begins to note proximal muscle cramps and weakness after exercise. She had noticed no symptoms when running the 100-meter dash for her college track team. Exam revealed her to be of short stature with proximal muscle weakness. Ophthalmologic exam revealed early signs of retinitis pigmentosa. She admits that both her mother and maternal grandmother developed similar symptoms. Which biochemical pathway would be disrupted?

    (A) glycolysis
    (B) glycogenolysis
    (C) Krebs cycle
    (D) electron transport chain
    (E) none

31. Which of the following cell types (shown in Figure 9.4) contains histamine and is responsible for the stimulation of parietal cell activity?

    (A) parietal cell
    (B) enterochromaffin-like cell (ECL)
    (C) mucous neck cell
    (D) D cell
    (E) eosinophil

32. The cholera toxin is produced by the organism *Vibrio cholera*, resulting in watery diarrhea. Which signaling cascade would be directly affected by the toxin?

    (A) adenylyl cyclase
    (B) phospholipase C

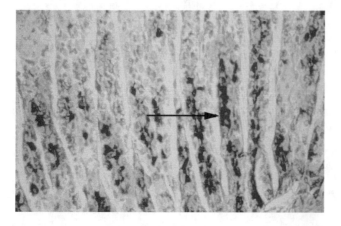

Figure 9.4

(C) protein kinase C
(D) protein kinase A
(E) protein kinase A and C

33. A 45-year-old woman presents to her physician with a history of pruritus. On examination, the patient appears to have jaundice and a mildly enlarged and tender liver. Laboratory studies reveal an elevation in alkaline phosphatase and bilirubin. Which of the following hepatic studies would be most appropriate for this patient?

    (A) serum ferritin
    (B) serum ceruloplasmin
    (C) serum antitrypsin
    (D) serum antimitochondrial antibodies (AMAs)
    (E) SGOT and SGPT

34. A 58-year-old man is admitted to the hospital due to severe thrombocytopenia. His only medication is ticlopidine, which he is on for a prior history of amaurosis fugax. On examination, he is noted to be febrile and confused. Skin reveals diffuse petechiae. Laboratory studies are significant for anemia, thrombocytopenia, and an elevated creatinine, but his coagulation profile (prothrombin time [PT] and activated partial thromboplastin time [aPTT]) is normal. A peripheral smear reveals the presence of numerous schistocytes. Of the choices given, what is the next best step?

    (A) platelet infusions
    (B) intravenous immunoglobulin (Ig) therapy
    (C) intravenous steroids
    (D) splenectomy
    (E) plasma exchange

35. Which of the following is characteristic of compartment syndrome of the lower leg?

    (A) pain relieved with aspirin
    (B) firm swelling of the calf
    (C) numbness of the foot
    (D) compartment pressure measurement less than 30 mmHg
    (E) absent distal pulses

36. Which of the following anatomic structures is involved in protection of the upper airway?

   (A) lower esophageal sphincter (LES)
   (B) epiglottis
   (C) uvula
   (D) tonsils
   (E) adenoids

37. What arthritic condition is associated with thick, coarse, dry skin lesions on the anterior aspect of the knees and the posterior aspect of the elbows?

   (A) osteoarthritis
   (B) psoriatic arthritis
   (C) septic arthritis
   (D) rheumatoid arthritis
   (E) Marie-Strümpell arthritis

38. What screening laboratory test would be consistent with a diagnosis of mitochondrial disorder?

   (A) increased serum lactate
   (B) reduced serum lactate
   (C) reduced serum glucose
   (D) increased serum carnitine
   (E) increased creatine phosphokinase (CPK)

39. A 72-year-old woman with small cell lung cancer comes to you complaining of progressive gait imbalance that worsens in the dark. She believes her symptoms began while receiving chemotherapy for her cancer. Your exam finds an absence of all reflexes with complete loss of proprioception and vibration sense. She has a positive Romberg test. You diagnose a polyneuropathy. She cannot remember which chemotherapeutic regimen she received, but you believe that you know. Which of the following did she receive?

   (A) vincristine
   (B) paclitaxel
   (C) cis-platinum
   (D) adriamycin
   (E) cyclophosphamide

40. Which neural pathway from brain to limb decussates at the level of the spinal cord?

   (A) corticospinal
   (B) reticulospinal
   (C) spinothalamic
   (D) dorsal column
   (E) spinocerebellar

41. An alpha motor neuron and all of the muscle cells it supplies is known as a

   (A) fasciculation
   (B) fibrillation
   (C) motor unit
   (D) compound motor action potential
   (E) muscle spindle

42. A 46-year-old man of Mediterranean descent is newly diagnosed with dermatitis herpetiformis. In anticipation of beginning dapsone therapy, a glucose-6-phosphate dehydrogenase (G6PD) deficiency is identified. He should avoid eating

   (A) asparagus
   (B) grapefruit
   (C) cranberries
   (D) fava beans
   (E) peanuts

43. A 12-year-old girl has a history of asthma and an acute flare of atopic dermatitis. Elaboration of which of the following cytokines is most characteristic of this situation?

   (A) interleukin-1
   (B) interleukin-2
   (C) interleukin-4
   (D) interferon-gamma
   (E) tumor necrosis factor-alpha

44. A 65-year-old man is scheduled to have scalp surgery for the removal of a large squamous cell carcinoma. Which of the following dietary supplements may inhibit platelet function, increasing the risk of excessive bleeding?

    (A) vitamin A
    (B) vitamin B
    (C) vitamin D
    (D) vitamin E
    (E) vitamin K

45. A 21-year-old man has male pattern baldness involving the vertex of his scalp. This condition has been associated with an increased risk of

    (A) coronary artery disease (CAD)
    (B) emphysema
    (C) gastritis
    (D) hypothyroidism
    (E) osteoporosis

Questions 46 through 50

46. Which of the following is best used in combination with another agent in premenopausal women with an intact uterus?

    (A) calcium
    (B) alendronate
    (C) calcitonin
    (D) estrogen
    (E) heparin

47. Which of the following must be taken in the morning while seated upright 30 minutes before breakfast?

    (A) calcium
    (B) alendronate
    (C) calcitonin
    (D) estrogen
    (E) heparin

48. Which of the following has an intranasal preparation?

    (A) calcium
    (B) alendronate
    (C) calcitonin
    (D) estrogen
    (E) heparin

49. Which of the following during long-term use can increase the risk of osteoporosis?

    (A) calcium
    (B) alendronate
    (C) calcitonin
    (D) estrogen
    (E) heparin

50. Which of the following has its absorption impeded by concomitant use of iron or caffeine?

    (A) calcium
    (B) alendronate
    (C) calcitonin
    (D) estrogen
    (E) heparin

Answers and Explanations

1. **(A)** Free fatty acids are converted to acetyl CoA, which cannot be converted to glucose. Glycerol, lactate, and amino acids can all participate in gluconeogenesis.

2. **(B)** The heart has very little ability to generate energy anaerobically. The tricarboxylic acid (TCA) cycle is operative in an aerobic state and results in nicotinamide adenine dinucleotide (NADH) and oxidative phosphorylation. With exercise, coronary arteriolar resistance decreases and allows increased coronary flow and increased O_2 consumption.

3. **(A)** There are no signs of heart failure present and the patient is very active making the diagnosis of dilated cardiomyopathy unlikely. The first heart sound has two components. M1 is related to closure of the mitral valve and T1 to closure of the tricuspid valve. Since the left ventricle begins contraction slightly before the right, it is possible to hear these components separately, particularly during expiration. A third heart sound is a low frequency diastolic heart sound and can be a normal finding in young, healthy adults. Abnormal heart sound splitting or murmur would be expected with the septal defects. Similarly, obstructive HCM should give rise to a murmur, and typically an S4 relates to diastolic stiffness.

4. **(C)** Propylthiouracil, a thioamide medication, is commonly used in patients with hyperthyroidism. This medication inhibits the iodination of tyrosyl residues as well as the coupling of iodotyrosines. It also inhibits the peripheral conversion of thyroxine (T_4) to triiodothyronine (T_3).

5. **(A)** Most of the mitotic activity in normal epidermis occurs in the basal cell layer.

6. **(D)** The spleen is an important aspect of the body's immune system. In particular, it is a major site of immunoglobulin M (IgM) production that is necessary for opsonization of encapsulated bacteria. Therefore, post-splenectomy sepsis can be fulminant, and immunization against encapsulated bacteria should be done, preferably prior to any elective splenectomy. The most common pathogen is *Streptococcus pneumoniae,* with a smaller incidence of postsplenectomy sepsis occurring with meningococcus and *Haemophilus.* Hepatitis B is a virus, and although it may be warranted in other situations, it is not indicated on the basis of the patient's asplenic status alone. Periodic repeat immunizations are felt to be prudent, although a specific time frame has not been clarified.

7. **(E)** CML is a marrow-derived blood dyscrasia of the granulocytic cell line in various stages of maturation. The Philadelphia chromosome results from the t9;22, which involves the movement of the majority of the ABL proto-oncogene from chromsome 9 to become contiguous with the 5' portion of the BCR gene on chromosome 22. This is associated with CML in 90% of cases and is also seen in Ph-positive acute lymphocytic leukemia (ALL).

8. **(C)** The desmosome is the intercellular bridge connecting keratinocytes.

9. **(D)** Further vascular studies are a waste of valuable time. Emergent closed reduction is in order and easily performed under IV sedation. Applying straight distal traction at the wrist will extend the elbow and lock the coronoid process of the ulna into the olecranon fossa of the distal humerus preventing reduction.

10. **(A)** Paget's disease is characterized by scattered areas of osteoblastic and lytic bone activity. Increased hydroxyproline urine levels indicate high bone turnover. Fibrous dysplasia is a benign bone process with areas of fibrous tissue surrounding small osteoid spicules resembling alphabet soup. Bence Jones proteins are secreted in the urine in multiple myeloma. Osteogenesis imperfecta is a genetically transmitted disease characterized by multiple infantile or childhood fractures. Affected children generally have blue sclerae.

11. **(B)** Plasmin, which is derived from plasminogen, degrades both fibrinogen and fibrin. Once the fibrin is cross-linked, the breakdown process is slower because plasmin cannot gain access to the stable fibrin polymer as readily as it can to the unstable non-cross-linked fibrin mesh.

12. **(C)** As *S. aureus* is the most common cause of bone infections, prophylactic IV cephalosporins are generally given prior to orthopedic surgeries. Hospital-acquired methicillin-resistant *S. aureus* is now very common and is resistant to commonly used cephalosporins such as cefazolin.

13. **(D)** This patient has had an acute inferior MI with right ventricular involvement. Hypotension is common with right ventricular involvement because of the inability of the damaged right ventricle to pump blood to the left side of the heart. Treatment with nitroglycerin reduces preload and would result in even more severe hypotension. Volume support is needed. The right coronary artery supplies the right ventricle and inferior myocardial wall in most people.

14. **(D)** Since ACTH is low, the source of the Cushing's is adrenal (either adrenal adenoma or carcinoma). Therefore, imaging of the adrenals is indicated.

15. **(A)** Osteoporosis treatment is aimed at decreasing osteoclastic activity with such compounds as bisphosphonates (alendronate) and hormonal manipulation (calcitonin and estrogen replacement). Osteomalacia is a metabolic bone disorder in which there is inadequate mineralization of newly formed osteoid. The childhood form is termed *rickets*.

16. **(D)** Growth hormone therapy promotes linear growth prior to the closure of the epiphyseal plates. Therefore, it would be ineffective in a 25-year-old man if used to increase height. Growth hormone in excess causes insulin resistance by impairing glucose uptake into cells. It increases protein synthesis by enhancing amino acid uptake, and increases the intestinal absorption of calcium. It acts on the liver to increase secretion of IGF-1, which mediates many of the effects of growth hormone.

17. **(A)** APML is characterized by prominent primary cytoplasmic granules as seen in normal promyelocytes. Due to the release of a procoagulant factor with thromboplastin, disseminated intravascular coagulation can occur. Leukemic blasts all have the characteristic translocation at 15;17. Recent studies have shown that the break point on chromosome 17 is an intron of the retinoic acid receptor alpha gene. This finding has allowed the treatment of APML with all-*trans* retinoic acid (ATRA), but its mechanism of action is still being elucidated.

18. **(B)** Trisomy 21 is the most common chromosomal disorder, occurring in 1 in 700 births overall. The most important risk factor is increasing maternal age, with an incidence of 1 in 30 in women over the age of 45 years.

Prenatal screening and diagnosis is possible and is routinely offered. Translocation of the long arm of chromosome 21 to chromosome 22 or 14 may occur and result in a triple dosage of chromosome 21 (robertsonian translocation). Therefore, Down syndrome may be familial as a result of a parent who is a carrier of a robertsonian translocation. This accounts for approximately 4% of cases of Down syndrome.

19. **(A)** Following fracture of diaphyseal bone, stem cells differentiate into chondroblasts and chondrocytes in the areas where fracture healing has outpaced the formation of capillaries. The chondrocytes form cartilage, which eventually becomes calcified. The enclosed chondrocytes die, and the cartilage is replaced with bone laid down by osteoblasts brought in by the advancing vascular tissue. The osteogenic layer of the periosteum lays down bone directly at the surface of the fracture site without an intermittent cartilage model.

20. **(B)** A serum cortisol of at least 20 µg/dL 60 minutes after cosyntropin is a normal response.

21. **(E)** Most standardized tests concerning the musculoskeletal system contain questions on the brachial plexus. The easiest way to handle these questions is to memorize the plexus in line-drawing form and reproduce it on the back of your test booklet at the start of the exam. Remember to include the five anterior root rami, three trunks, six divisions, three cords, and six terminal branches.

22. **(C)** After the diagnosis of adrenal insufficiency is made based on the cosyntropin stimulation test, ACTH level is drawn to identify the etiology: A high level indicates primary (adrenal) insufficiency; a low/normal level indicates secondary (pituitary) insufficiency.

23. **(D)** The basal cells are attached to the subepidermal basement membrane zone by modified desmosomes called hemidesmosomes.

24. **(B)** The most likely site of iron deficiency is the gastrointestinal tract, especially with the presence of occult blood in the stools. The next most appropriate examination would be an upper endoscopy. A bone marrow aspirate would not be helpful to identify the source of GI blood loss. A bleeding scan is rarely positive unless the bleeding is active. A barium enema would have a low sensitivity to identify a source for iron deficiency given that the colonoscopy was negative.

25. **(D)** With left ventricular hypertrophy, resting abnormalities are common and will interfere with the ability to diagnose changes on the ECG during exercise. Coronary arteriography should be undertaken only after ischemia has been demonstrated. A resting echocardiogram will give functional information, but a stress echocardiogram will give dynamic functional information about heart muscle function. Development of wall motion abnormalities during exercise strongly suggests ischemia and coronary artery disease.

26. **(E)** Answers A through D are typical of rheumatoid arthritis (RA). First-line drugs used in the treatment of RA are cortisone and NSAIDs. Second-line drugs include gold, hydrochloroquine, and older chemotherapeutic agents such as methotrexate.

27. **(C)** According to Wolff's law, bone remodels to compressive forces. Trabeculae form and align themselves to the compressive lines of stress. All of the other choices are true statements about the properties of bone.

28. **(E)** Cushing's disease is caused by excess ACTH secretion by the pituitary gland and is characterized by high serum and urine cortisol levels and by normal to high ACTH levels. Features may include wide, purplish abdominal striae; fragile skin; poor wound healing; muscle weakness; and osteopenia/osteoporosis.

29. **(A)** Insulin Lispro has a duration of action of 3 to 4 hours. Regular insulin lasts 5 to 7

hours, NPH lasts 18 to 24 hours, and Ultra-lente lasts 25 to 36 hours.

30. **(D)** The majority of mitochondrial disorders follow maternal inheritance, as children receive all of their mitochondria from the mother. There are often enzymatic abnormalities within the electron transport chain.

31. **(B)** The parietal cell contains the H^+,K^+ ATPase and is responsible for the release of gastric acid into the stomach. The ECL cell contains histamine, which stimulates the secretion of acid by the parietal cell. The figure demonstrates staining of the ECL cell in the stomach. The mucous neck cell of the stomach is responsible for protecting the stomach against acid injury. The D cell of the stomach contains somatostatin that has an inhibitory effect on the release of gastric acid.

32. **(A)** The cholera toxin specifically stimulates intestinal adenylyl cyclase, resulting in diarrhea. The toxin would not influence the other signaling pathways listed.

33. **(D)** In patients with primary biliary cirrhosis (PBC), the serum alkaline phosphatase concentration is almost always elevated, whereas the serum levels of aminotransferases may be normal or slightly elevated. Early in the course of the disease, the serum bilirubin concentration is usually normal but becomes elevated in most patients as the disease progresses resulting in an icteric state and manifested by pruritus. AMA is the laboratory hallmark for the diagnosis of PBC. An elevated serum ferritin level is associated with hemochromatosis. Serum antitrypsin levels are important in the evaluation of patients suspected of having antitrypsin deficiency.

34. **(E)** The clinical picture is that of thrombotic thrombocytopenic purpura (TTP). The hallmark of this diagnosis depends on the presence of evidence for microangiopathic hemolysis. This is generally evident on a peripheral smear with evidence of red cell fragments or schistocytes. The clinical pentad is that of fever, renal dysfunction, neurologic changes, thrombocytopenia, and evidence of microangiopathic hemolysis. This syndrome is closely related to the hemolytic–uremic syndrome (HUS), and they are sometimes distinguished from each other on the basis of clinical features. However, it appears that TTP is specifically related to an inherited or acquired defect in the activity of a protease that cleaves the unusually large von Willebrand factor multimers. (In children, the development of HUS has been closely linked to the release of a shiga toxin from patients with dysentery due to *E. coli* O157:H7.) Disseminated intravascular coagulation (DIC) may produce a similar picture to TTP, but unlike TTP, the coagulation cascade is activated and consumption of coagulation factors typically leads to prolongation of the PT and the aPTT in DIC. The primary mode of therapy in TTP is plasma exchange. The benefits in particular seem to be associated with the volume of plasma infused. The theoretical benefit of this therapy may be a result of repleting the large von Willebrand multimer protease that is deficient in the patient with TTP.

35. **(B)** In an acute compartment syndrome, muscle swelling within a tight fascial covering leads to an increase in compartment pressure that can overcome small vessel pressures. This leads to loss of muscle perfusion and, therefore, muscle necrosis. Distal pulses are rarely absent. Some numbness in the foot may be present, but often a neurologic exam is normal. Pain is usually "out of proportion" to findings. Passive flexion–extension of the toes is very painful.

36. **(B)** The tonsils and uvula have no protective role in the upper airway. Reflexes involving the larynx, epiglottis, and arytenoids are involved in protecting the upper airway during swallowing. Impairments of the reflex can result in aspiration.

37. **(B)** Psoriatic arthritis is a seronegative arthritis characterized by skin lesions, involvement of the cervical spine in 70%, and frequent arthritic involvement of the hip.

38. **(A)** Due to "backup" of substrate entering the Krebs cycle, there is usually elevation in both serum pyruvate and lactate.

39. **(C)** Platinum agents commonly cause a pure large-fiber sensory neuropathy. The symptoms worsen with each treatment and then improve. Most patients obtain substantial improvement after cessation of the treatment. Vincristine causes a pure small-fiber sensory neuropathy, while paclitaxel predominantly affects small sensory fibers but can affect motor fibers as well.

40. **(C)** The spinothalamic pathway crosses one to two levels above its dermatomal representation. The proprioceptive/vibratory pathways that ultimately become the dorsal columns cross as the medial lemniscus at the brain stem, and the lateral corticospinal tracts cross at the pyramids within the medulla (though 15% of corticospinal fibers do not not cross and continue as the anterior corticospinal tract). The cerebellar pathways cross twice, allowing for an ipsilateral representation of signs and symptoms of a cerebellar lesion.

41. **(C)** The number of motor units in a particular muscle and their size (number of muscle cells per motor neuron) is dependent on the function of the muscle. For instance, a paraspinus muscle with limited demands may have few motor units, each of which has many muscle cells. In contrast, an extraocular muscle, which needs to make frequent small movements, may have the highest number of motor units composed of relatively few muscle cells. Individual motor units may be visualized during electromyography.

42. **(D)** G6PD deficiency generally does not produce any symptoms unless red blood cells are subjected to oxidative stress resulting in hemolytic anemia. Various drugs including sulfonamides have been reported to precipitate hemolytic anemia in patients with G6PD deficiency. Of the food choices, only fava beans have been shown in some individuals to cause oxidative injury.

43. **(C)** T-helper-2 cells produce a cytokine profile that activates humoral immunity. This clinical scenario would elicit a humoral immune response mediated by T-helper-2 cells such as interleukin-4. The other choices are associated with a T-helper-1 or cell-mediated immune response.

44. **(D)** Vitamin E, alpha-tocopherol, is known to inhibit platelet aggregation and adhesion. The other vitamins do not impact platelets.

45. **(A)** Male pattern baldness developing at a young age involving the vertex of the scalp has been associated with an increased risk of CAD.

46–50. **(46-D, 47-B, 48-C, 49-E, 50-A)** Estrogen given without progesterone in a patient with an intact uterus will increase the risk of endometrial cancer and cannot be given. Estrogen and progesterone need to be given in combination unless the patient has had a hysterectomy. Alendronate and the other bisphosphonates have a high risk of pill esophagitis and need to be taken first thing in the morning on an empty stomach and the patient must remain upright. Calcitonin comes in an intranasal preparation and is used to prevent or treat osteoporosis. Heparin will increase the risk of osteoporosis if used long term. Finally, calcium is not absorbed effectively if taken with iron or caffeine.

Practice Test 10
Questions

DIRECTIONS (Questions 1 through 50): Each of the numbered items or incomplete statements in this section is followed by answers or by completions of the statement. Select the ONE lettered answer or completion that is BEST in each case.

1. Which of the following is the primary component of the extracellular matrix of articular cartilage?

   (A) water
   (B) collagen
   (C) keratin sulfate
   (D) chondroitin sulfate
   (E) fibrous bone

2. Your patient with meningitis is found to have a normal cerebrospinal fluid (CSF) glucose. You suspect which of the following?

   (A) tuberculous meningitis
   (B) pneumococcal meningitis
   (C) carcinomatous meningitis
   (D) syphilitic meningitis
   (E) cryptococcal meningitis

3. The embryologic precursors of the uterus, tubes, cervix, and upper vagina are the

   (A) müllerian ducts
   (B) wolffian ducts
   (C) oogonium
   (D) endodermic wall of the primitive gut
   (E) oocyte

4. Regarding the P wave on the electrocardiogram (ECG), which of the following is true?

   (A) The P wave corresponds with depolarization of the His-Purkinje system.

   (B) The P wave is inscribed after depolarization of the sinoatrial (SA) node.
   (C) The P wave reflects atrial contraction.
   (D) The P wave results from depolarization of pacemaker cells within the sinus node.
   (E) The P wave is always present.

5. A true statement about a phenotypical female with a normally developed lower vagina and absent upper vagina and uterus is that

   (A) she also probably has no ovaries
   (B) her karyotype is 46,XY
   (C) she has Rokitansky-Kuster-Hauser syndrome
   (D) she probably has Klinefelter syndrome
   (E) her upper vagina is enlarged

6. A very high CSF protein in the absence of CSF white cells is found in

   (A) Lyme disease
   (B) Guillain-Barré syndrome
   (C) neurosyphilis
   (D) multiple sclerosis
   (E) neurosarcoidosis

7. A 65-year-old man is admitted with a myocardial infarction (MI). His lipid profile shows a cholesterol of 280 mg/dL. The high-density lipoprotein (HDL) level was 30 mg/dL and the triglyceride level was 320 mg/dL. What is his low-density lipoprotein (LDL) level?

   (A) 250 mg/dL
   (B) 186 mg/dL
   (C) 226 mg/dL
   (D) 216 mg/dL
   (E) 157 mg/dL

8. A 1-cm injury of articular cartilage extending into subchondral bone

   (A) repairs with fibrous scar tissue
   (B) repairs with normal articular hyaline cartilage
   (C) repairs with an inferior fibrocartilage-like material
   (D) fills in with bone leading to post-traumatic arthritis
   (E) will not repeat itself

9. A 20-year-old man is involved in a knife fight. He is transported to the emergency department (ED) and arrives with a blood pressure of 80/60, a pulse of 110 bpm, and a respiratory rate of 18. He is in and out of consciousness on arrival. A chest wound to the left of the sternum is noted immediately. Which of the following is the most likely diagnosis?

   (A) cardiac tamponade
   (B) ruptured pulmonary artery
   (C) pneumothorax
   (D) perforation of the aorta
   (E) perforation of the left ventricle

10. A 55-year-old man is referred to you for evaluation of chronic flushing that occurs at rest and is not associated with diet. The physical examination is otherwise unremarkable. A presumptive diagnosis of carcinoid syndrome can be made with elevations of which of the following laboratory tests?

    (A) serum bilirubin
    (B) serum porphyrins
    (C) urine 5-HIAA (hydroxyindoleacetic acid)
    (D) urine serotonin
    (E) serum epinephrine

11. Which of the following is part of the spinal cord gray matter and thought to be spared in multiple sclerosis (MS)?

    (A) corticospinal tract
    (B) dorsal column
    (C) anterior horn cell

    (D) internal capsule
    (E) corpus callosum

12. A patient is found to have an autoimmune adrenalitis as the cause of her adrenal insufficiency. You would treat her with

    (A) hydrocortisone
    (B) fludrocortisone
    (C) prednisone
    (D) hydrocortisone and fludrocortisone
    (E) hydrocortisone and prednisone

13. Which of the following statements concerning human skeletal muscle is true?

    (A) Low-tension, high-repetition training of long duration causes hypertrophy of fast-twitch, glycolytic fibers.
    (B) High-tension, low-repetition training causes hypertrophy of slow-twitch, oxidative fibers.
    (C) Endurance training causes hypertrophy of slow-twitch fibers with high aerobic capacity.
    (D) Muscle mass remains constant until age 60, then rapidly begins to decline.
    (E) Muscle mass itself does not alter with age.

14. A girl with stage 4 Tanner development exhibits

    (A) no breast development
    (B) very sparse pubic hair over labia majora only
    (C) regular menstrual cycles
    (D) breast enlargement with areolae above breast contour
    (E) irregular menstrual cycles

15. A 70-year-old man with a history of a berry aneurysm at the bifurcation of the anterior communicating artery presents to the ED with a headache and is diagnosed with a hemorrhagic cerebrovascular accident (CVA) via computed tomographic (CT) scan. Which of the following abnormalities is he most likely to have?

(A) Goodpasture's syndrome

(B) Reiter's syndrome

(C) adult polycystic kidney disease

(D) sarcoidosis

(E) Pancoast tumor

16. A 37-year-old man with a 10-year history of ulcerative colitis presents to his physician with a history of fever, right upper quadrant pain, and jaundice. An abdominal ultrasound and CT examination reveal dilated bile ducts and no evidence of cholelithiasis. An endoscopic retrograde cholangiopancreatography (ERCP) is performed, which shows multiple strictures involving the common bile duct. What is the most likely diagnosis for this patient?

(A) hepatocellular carcinoma

(B) sclerosing cholangitis

(C) primary biliary cirrhosis

(D) choledocholithiasis

(E) hepatorenal syndrome

17. A 24-year-old woman from Pennsylvania presents with fatigue, weight gain, dry skin, and irregular periods. Her family history is significant for a mother who has a "thyroid problem." On physical exam, she has a diffuse, nontender goiter, and her ankle reflexes exhibit a delayed relaxation phase. She is found to have a thyroid-stimulating hormone (TSH) of 25 µU/mL (normal: 0.4–4.8) and a free thyroxine (T_4) of 0.4 ng/dL (normal: 0.7–1.6). Antithyroid peroxidase antibodies are positive. What is the most likely cause of her hypothyroidism?

(A) iodine deficiency

(B) chronic lymphocytic thyroiditis (Hashimoto's thyroiditis)

(C) granulomatous thyroiditis (subacute thyroiditis)

(D) Graves' disease

(E) pituitary hypofunction

18. Iron-deficiency anemia is caused most often by

(A) liver disease

(B) peptic ulcer disease

(C) renal failure

(D) pancreatitis

(E) cardiomyopathy

19. What is the most common cause of skin cancer?

(A) viral infection

(B) ultraviolet radiation exposure

(C) infrared radiation exposure

(D) arsenic exposure

(E) x-ray exposure

20. Which of the following coagulation factors is either reduced or absent in classic hemophilia (hemophilia A)?

(A) factor I

(B) factor X

(C) factor III

(D) factor XIII

(E) factor VIII

21. Which of the following peptides is secreted from the pancreatic B cell in equimolar amounts with insulin?

(A) preproinsulin

(B) amylin (islet amyloid polypeptide)

(C) pancreatic polypeptide

(D) proinsulin

(E) C-peptide

Questions 22 through 24

Refer to Figure 10.1 for questions 22 through 24.

22. A 47-year-old nurse with a history of asthma refractory to medical treatment seeks a second opinion regarding her dyspnea. It is episodic and occurs in stressful or anxiety-provoking situations. She develops audible wheezing. Prior pulmonary function tests and methacholine challenge tests have been negative. Her medical history is otherwise significant for depression and an anxiety disorder. She returns during an acute attack, and a fiberoptic laryngoscopy reveals paradoxical closure of her vocal cords during inspiration. A diagnosis of paradoxical vocal cord dysfunction is made. If a pulmonary function test is performed on this patient during an acute attack, what is the likely shape of her flow-volume curve in Figure 10.1?

    (A) A
    (B) B
    (C) C
    (D) D
    (E) circular without any peak

23. A 60-year-old woman has had progressive dyspnea and now hemoptysis. As part of her evaluation, a bronchscopy is performed revealing a mass lesion 3 cm above the carina causing luminal narrowing. What is likely to be the shape of the flow-volume curve in this patient?

    (A) A
    (B) B
    (C) C
    (D) D
    (E) circular without any peak

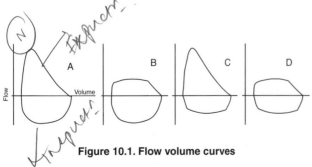

Figure 10.1. Flow volume curves

24. A 38-year-old man presents for an elective surgery requiring general anesthesia. Despite good visualization of the vocal cords, the anesthesiologist is unable to pass an endotracheal tube. Fiberoptic bronchoscopy suggests an area of severe tracheal stenosis distal to the larynx. Further history confirms increasing dyspnea and wheezing with a childhood illness that required prolonged intubation and mechanical ventilation. What is the likely shape of the flow-volume curve for this patient?

    (A) A
    (B) B
    (C) C
    (D) D
    (E) circular without any peak

25. A patient who was recently diagnosed with a right-sided stroke involving the posterior inferior cerebellar artery presents with difficulty in swallowing and new-onset hoarseness. Which of the following cranial nerves is likely to be involved?

    (A) CN III
    (B) CN V
    (C) CN VII
    (D) CN IX
    (E) CN II

26. Functional bowel disease may be caused by which of the following?

    (A) infection
    (B) hyperalgesia
    (C) aging
    (D) antibiotics
    (E) antispasmodics

27. Gastrin is a gastrointestinal hormone associated with

    (A) gastric motility
    (B) gastric acid secretion
    (C) intestinal motility
    (D) intestinal secretion
    (E) esophageal motility

28. Which of the following disease states has a genetic basis?

    (A) familial adenomatous polyposis (FAP)
    (B) sporadic adenomas
    (C) colon cancer
    (D) gastric cancer
    (E) hyperplastic colonic polyps

29. Wilson's disease is characterized by an abnormal metabolism with

    (A) elevated iron stores
    (B) elevated copper stores
    (C) inability to metabolize fructose
    (D) inability to metabolize lactose
    (E) elevated zinc

30. Short-bowel syndrome is associated with

    (A) nausea and vomiting
    (B) gastroparesis
    (C) diarrhea and intestinal malabsorption
    (D) thrombosis of the mesenteric vessels
    (E) persisting constipation

31. The bone with the highest rate of fracture nonunion is the

    (A) femur
    (B) carpal scaphoid
    (C) humerus
    (D) radius
    (E) tibia

32. The initial sign of puberty in most (85% to 90%) of girls is

    (A) growth of axillary hair
    (B) development of breast buds
    (C) growth of pubic hair
    (D) onset of menses
    (E) onset of excessive use of the telephone

33. Five patients are seen during grand rounds, each representing one of the following conditions. You tell one patient that his condition will not transform into acute leukemia. Which one?

    (A) patient 1 with chronic lymphocytic leukemia (CLL)
    (B) patient 2 with myelofibrosis
    (C) patient 3 with Hodgkin's lymphoma
    (D) patient 4 with polycythemia vera
    (E) patient 5 with chronic myelogenous leukemia (CML)

34. Which of the following test results establishes a diagnosis of diabetes mellitus?

    (A) fasting plasma glucose at least 126 mg/dL
    (B) 2-hour glucose greater than 140 mg/dL during an oral glucose tolerance test
    (C) random plasma glucose greater than 140 mg/dL
    (D) Hb_{A1c} (glycohemoglobin A1c) greater than 6.0%
    (E) excessive craving for sugar

35. Aspirin affects the function of cyclooxygenase, resulting in which of the following?

    (A) inhibition of platelet function, resulting in an increased bleeding time
    (B) blocked transformation of vitamin K in the liver, which inhibits the production of factors II, VII, IX, and X
    (C) enhanced ability of antithrombin III to inhibit factors thrombin, IX-a, and X-a, increasing the partial thromboplastin time (PTT)
    (D) inhibition of factors X-a and II-a
    (E) reduced cell "clumping"

36. The most common form of atrial septal defect (ASD) is

    (A) ostium primum
    (B) sinus venosus
    (C) muscular septal
    (D) ostium secundum
    (E) ostium venosus

37. Most of the glucose in the kidney is reabsorbed in the

   (A) distal convoluted tubule
   (B) proximal convoluted tubule
   (C) thin descending limb of the loop of Henle
   (D) collecting tubule
   (E) thick ascending limb of the loop of Henle

38. You see a 45-year-old woman with resistant hypertension. She is on amlodipine, atenolol, and furosemide. You decide to screen her for primary hyperaldosteronism. What would you do?

   (A) CT scan of the adrenals
   (B) adrenal vein sampling
   (C) plasma aldosterone and renin
   (D) plasma aldosterone after 1 mg dexamethasone
   (E) serum potassium

39. The uterine artery arises from the

   (A) aorta
   (B) anterior branch of the hypogastric artery
   (C) posterior branch of the hypogastric artery
   (D) common iliac artery
   (E) inguinal artery

40. A 56-year-old woman with a history of kidney stones is found to have an elevated calcium level and decreased phosphorus level on routine blood work. Her 24-hour urine calcium is elevated. She has no significant complaints and her physical exam is unremarkable. What is the most likely primary hormone excess involved?

   (A) 25-hydroxyvitamin D
   (B) parathyroid hormone (PTH)
   (C) calcitonin
   (D) 1,25-dihydroxyvitamin D
   (E) levothyroxine (T_4)

41. Increased filling pressures, decreased cardiac output (CO), and increased systemic vascular resistance (SVR) are noted with

   (A) pulmonary embolism (PE)
   (B) hypovolemic shock
   (C) septic shock
   (D) cardiogenic shock
   (E) normal vasculature

42. Which factor will be unaltered in a state of vitamin K deficiency?

   (A) prothrombin (factor II)
   (B) factor V
   (C) factor VII
   (D) factor IX
   (E) factor X

43. Which of the following medications might be implicated in causing constipation in an elderly patient?

   (A) barbiturates
   (B) opioid narcotics
   (C) H_2 receptor antagonists
   (D) proton pump inhibitors (PPIs)
   (E) Mylanta

44. Which of the following is characteristic of patients with polycythemia vera?

   (A) reduced hematocrit
   (B) elevated erythropoietin level
   (C) elevated platelet count
   (D) younger age
   (E) less-than-average chance of stroke or MI

45. A positive secretin test would be useful in the diagnosis of

   (A) Zollinger-Ellison syndrome
   (B) carcinoid syndrome
   (C) Ménétrier's disease
   (D) peptic ulcer disease
   (E) GERD

46. A 30-year-old woman has had increasing dyspnea, weight loss, diarrhea, and palpitations. Examination reveals a large, grossly visible multinodular goiter. If the goiter is compromising her airways and causing her dyspnea, what is likely to be the shape of her flow-volume curve (Figure 10.2)?

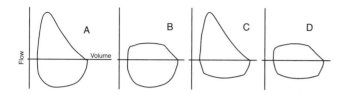

Figure 10.2

(A) A

(B) B

(C) C

(D) a pattern like A but more peaked

(E) a pattern like C but more peaked

47. What is the characteristic rash of Lyme disease?

(A) erythema marginatum

(B) erythema migrans

(C) erythema gyratum repens

(D) erythema nodosum

(E) erythema annulare centrifugum

48. A 46-year-old man undergoes surgery for a 3-cm pituitary adenoma. Several hours postoperatively, he develops severe thirst and urinary frequency, with a urine output of 5 liters in 12 hours. His serum sodium is 155 mmol/L (normal: 135–145 mmol/L), serum osmolality 320 mOsm/kg H_2O (normal: 275–290 mOsm/kg H_2O), and urine specific gravity 1.002 (range: 1.002–1.028). What is the most likely diagnosis?

(A) diabetes insipidus (impaired antidiuretic hormone [ADH] secretion)

(B) diabetes mellitus

(C) hyperthyroidism

(D) syndrome of inappropriate ADH secretion (SIADH)

(E) hypoglycemia

49. A 16-year-old girl is referred to you for amenorrhea and hirsutism. You suspect congenital adrenal hyperplasia (CAH). Which of the following enzyme deficiencies is the most common cause of CAH?

(A) 11β-hydroxylase

(B) 21α-hydroxylase

(C) 17α-hydroxylase

(D) 3β-hydroxysteroid dehydrogenase

(E) amylase deficiency

50. A 25-year-old patient with headache, fever, and nuchal rigidity presents to the ED and bacterial meningitis is suspected. This hospital has had isolates of *Streptococcus pneumoniae* that show resistance to beta-lactam antibiotics. The empiric antibiotic regimen should be

(A) ceftriaxone 2 g IV q 24 hours

(B) ceftriaxone 2 g IV q 12 hours and vancomycin

(C) acyclovir only

(D) ampicillin only

(E) penicillin VK 250 mg qid PO

Answers and Explanations

1. **(A)** The extracellular matrix is 65% to 80% water. The predominant collagen is type II. The aggrecan proteoglycan molecule comprises many glycosaminoglycan chains of keratin sulfate and chondroitin sulfate that carry a predominant negative charge. This is responsible for the high water content and, therefore, the deformability of articular cartilage.

2. **(D)** The CSF glucose is typically normal in spirochetal infections such as syphilis and Lyme disease and in most viral meningitides, although herpes simplex can have a mild reduction. The CSF glucose is low in choices A, B, C, and E.

3. **(A)** The wolffian ducts are the precursors of the male structures. *Oogonium* is the term applied to the primitive oocyte. The primitive germ cells migrate from the endodermic wall of the primitive gut in early embryonic life.

4. **(B)** The P wave is inscribed only after depolarization of the SA node. The mechanical activity follows the depolarization.

5. **(C)** Partial müllerian aplasia or Rokitansky-Kuster-Hauser syndrome causes congenital absence of the upper vagina. These patients usually have normal ovaries and have a 46,XX karyotype. Patients with Klinefelter syndrome have a 47,XXY karyotype and are phenotypically males, though they have azoospermia and may have gynecomastia.

6. **(B)** All of the other choices manifest a CSF monocytic pleocytosis. The high protein seen in Guillain-Barré syndrome arises due to demyelination of the motor roots, which pass through spinal fluid as they exit the spinal canal. This high protein count may not be seen for several days after onset of the disease.

7. **(B)** The LDL is typically calculated rather than measured. The formula is: LDL = cholesterol – HDL – triglyceride/5.

8. **(C)** Injuries extending into subchondral bone will repair with fibrocartilage, which is inferior to normal articular cartilage but better than scar tissue. This is the reason that drilling into bleeding subchondral bone is performed arthroscopically for osteochondral and other significant articular cartilage injuries.

9. **(A)** Anatomically, the right ventricle is behind the sternum and extends to the left of the sternum. The left ventricle is located further to the left of the sternum. The aorta is significantly posterior. The lung is displaced by the heart to the left of the sternum.

10. **(C)** The most sensitive test for the establishment of a diagnosis of carcinoid syndrome is the 24-hour urinary 5-HIAA level. Serum serotonin, although useful, is not the most sensitive and specific study given that serum serotonin levels are greatly influenced by ingestion of certain foods such as tomatoes and nuts. Serum bilirubin levels are not affected by carcinoid syndrome, and serum porphyrin levels are generally normal.

11. **(C)** All of the other options are myelinated neuronal tracts that make up white matter.

The anterior horn cell is part of spinal cord gray matter that was thought to be relatively spared in MS. More attention is being paid to the early axonal injury and neuronal damage seen pathologically in patients with more severe MS and its relationship to long-term disability.

12. (D) Patients with primary adrenal insufficiency need glucocorticoid and mineralocorticoid replacement.

13. (C) Muscle mass begins to decline at age 25, and the rate of this decline increases at age 50. Low-tension, high-repetition training of long duration increases capillary density and the concentration of mitochondria, increasing the capability of oxidative metabolism. This causes hypertrophy of slow-twitch, oxidative fibers. High-tension, low-repetition training emphasizes development of muscle strength and power. Hypertrophy of fast-twitch glycolytic fibers occurs.

14. (D) Presence or absence of menses is not part of Tanner staging. Stage 4 Tanner development describes breast development as in choice D and adult character of pubic hair that has not yet spread laterally from the mons to lateral upper thighs.

15. (C) There exists a strong correlation between adult polycystic kidney disease and berry aneurysms of the circle of Willis. Berry aneurysm ruptures can be associated with a hemorrhagic CVA, which can present as a headache or neurologic deficit.

16. (B) The case in question points to a diagnosis of primary sclerosing cholangitis (PSC). The diagnosis of PSC is established by the demonstration of multifocal stricturing and dilation of intrahepatic and/or extrahepatic bile ducts during a cholangiographic examination (i.e., ERCP). Although strictures can occur in any part of the biliary tree, the majority occur distally. Epidemiologically, the majority of cases have underlying ulcerative colitis; the prevalence may be as high as 90%. The cholangiographic findings are not suggestive of hepatocellular carcinoma, which occurs in patients with underlying cirrhosis and presents as a hepatic mass. Primary biliary cirrhosis is not associated with ulcerative colitis and generally spares the extrahepatic biliary tree. Although choledocholithiasis is more common in patients with ulcerative colitis, it does not produce strictures of the common bile duct. In addition, cholelithiasis in this case was excluded on ultrasonographic examination.

17. (B) Chronic lymphocytic thyroiditis is the most common cause of hypothyroidism in the United States. There is often a family history of autoimmune thyroid dysfunction. Physical exam will often reveal a goiter; dry, puffy skin; and a delayed reflex relaxation phase. Antithyroid antibodies are positive in almost 97% of patients. Iodine deficiency is rarely a cause of hypothyroidism in the United States but can be seen in developing countries. Hypothyroidism may occur in the late phase of subacute thyroiditis, but this disorder is much less common than Hashimoto's thyroiditis and usually associated with neck pain. Graves' disease typically presents with symptoms of hyperthyroidism such as weight loss, tremors, and tachycardia. In pituitary hypothyroidism, the TSH is normal to decreased rather than elevated.

18. (B) Peptic ulcers lead to chronic blood loss and thus loss of iron. Although severe liver disease can cause gastrointestinal bleeding through ruptured varices, the bleeding is generally acute rather than chronic. The anemia of renal failure is due to toxic damage to the bone marrow, and iron stores thus remain normal. Cardiomyopathy and pancreatitis are not associated with anemia in general.

19. (B) The most common cause of skin cancer is ultraviolet radiation, which is a complete carcinogen.

20. (E) The coagulation factor VIII complex is under the control of the X chromosome and is reduced or absent in classic hemophilia.

Factor VIII is also reduced in von Willebrand's disease, which is an autosomal-dominant disorder characterized by an abnormality in the plasma protein von Willebrand's factor, which is part of the VIII complex.

21. **(E)**   Proinsulin is cleaved by converting enzymes to form insulin and C-peptide, both of which are secreted from the pancreas in equimolar quantities. Preproinsulin is synthesized by the human insulin gene on chromosome 11 and is immediately cleaved to form proinsulin. Amylin, or islet amyloid polypeptide, is stored in the B cell with insulin, but in a ratio of 1 molecule of amylin to 100 molecules of insulin. Pancreatic polypeptide is secreted from pancreatic F cells.

22. **(C)**   Paradoxical vocal cord dysfunction results in the paradoxical closure of vocal cords during inspiration. The stridor is often mistaken for wheezing, and the disorder is thought to be a conversion disorder. The closing of the vocal cords during inspiration causes limitation of flow during forced inspiration and therefore is marked by truncation of the inspiratory phase of the flow-volume curve. This is an example of a variable extrathoracic obstruction. More typically, a lesion in the extrathoracic upper airways will produce this picture. The flow limitation occurs only during inspiration, as the luminal pressure is lower than atmospheric pressure during inspiration, consequently causing a narrowing. During expiration, the luminal pressure is higher and therefore causes the airways to expand even at the site of the lesion, allowing normal flows. Extrathoracic tracheomalacia would be another example of a cause of variable extrathoracic obstruction.

23. **(B)**   In this situation, the lesion is in the intrathoracic upper airways. With inspiration, negative intrathoracic pressures are generated outside of the trachea. Therefore, any luminal narrowing caused by the lesion will open further with forced inspiration and therefore inspiratory flows are likely to be preserved. However, during forced expiration, the intrathoracic pressure outside the trachea is greater than the pressure within

the trachea, accentuating any flow limitations at the site of the lesion. This will be seen as a truncation of the forced expiratory flow-volume curve while the forced inspiratory phase is preserved. This is referred to as variable intrathoracic obstruction.

24. **(D)**   This is an example of a fixed upper airway obstruction. Tracheal stenosis is a fixed lesion that will not vary with pressure gradients that are created during forced inspiration or expiration. If the stenosis is narrow enough to compromise air flow, it should then be reflected in both phases of the flow-volume curve, with truncation during both forced inspiration and forced expiration.

25. **(D)**   The glossopharyngeal nerve is involved with nerve supply to the upper aerodigestive tract, and dysfunction can be seen in bulbar strokes, causing dysphagia and speech abnormalities.

26. **(B)**   Functional bowel disease may be caused by visceral hyperalgesia and is not related to the presence of infection. Aging and medications would not be associated with the development of functional bowel disease.

27. **(B)**   Gastrin is released by the gastric G cell in response to food stimulation, which stimulates histamine release from the gastric enterochromaffin-like (ECL) cell resulting in gastric acid secretion. Gastrin is not associated with motility or intestinal secretion.

28. **(A)**   Choices B, C, and D do not have a genetic basis for acquiring the disease. Patients with FAP have a predisposition to develop multiple colonic polyps and a significant risk for the development of colorectal cancers.

29. **(B)**   Patients with Wilson's disease have elevated stores of copper and not iron. Patients with Wilson's disease do not have an inability to metabolize either fructose or lactose.

30. **(C)**   Intestinal malabsorption can result from intestinal surgery, resulting in a blind loop, which predisposes to the proliferation of bacteria. This may result in malabsorption and

diarrhea. Gastroparesis is not generally associated with short-bowel syndrome. Nausea and vomiting are not hallmark symptoms in patients with short bowel syndrome. Mesenteric thrombosis is a medical emergency and would result in more severe symptoms indicative of a surgical abdomen.

31. **(E)** Of the bones listed, the tibia has the poorest blood supply.

32. **(B)** In African-American girls, pubic hair is slightly more often the initial sign of development, and this can be a normal variant in white girls as well.

33. **(C)** Polycythemia vera and myelofibrosis are chronic conditions involving dysplastic marrow, thus carrying a risk of leukemia. Both CML and CLL have the ability to transform to acute leukemia, although this occurs more with CML than CLL. Although some lymphomas, especially the small cleaved cells, can undergo leukemic transformation, Hodgkin's disease is not known to do so. However, the treatment for Hodgkin's disease does increase long-term risk for a secondary leukemia potential.

34. **(A)** The criteria for a diagnosis of diabetes mellitus include a fasting plasma glucose at least 126 mg/dL, a 2-hour glucose at least 200 mg/dL during an oral glucose tolerance test, or a random plasma glucose at least 200 mg/dL associated with symptoms of diabetes (polyuria, polydipsia, or weight loss). An Hb_{A1c} is not sufficiently sensitive to detect impaired glucose tolerance and is used primarily to monitor the effectiveness of treatment in patients with diabetes.

35. **(A)** Aspirin affects platelet aggregation, resulting in a prolonged bleeding time. Bleeding time can be affected by a single aspirin tablet for up to 14 days.

36. **(D)** The septum secundum forms on the right side of the septum primum and covers the ostium secundum. The foramen ovale is formed in this way. Faulty development of the septum secundum results in the most

common type of ASD (ostium secundum defect).

37. **(B)** Most of the glucose, amino acids, bicarbonate, water, and sodium of the filtrate are reabsorbed in the proximal convoluted tubule.

38. **(C)** A useful screening test for primary hyperaldosteronism is a plasma aldosterone-to-renin ratio. When diagnosis is confirmed, CT scan of the adrenals is done. If the CT scan is not conclusive, then adrenal vein sampling is performed. Serum potassium can be normal in up to 20% of patients with hyperaldosteronism. The test in choice D does not exist.

39. **(A)** This anatomic fact is important when performing hypogastric artery ligation to control postpartum hemorrhage.

40. **(B)** PTH causes increased serum calcium levels by increasing calcium absorption in the kidney, increasing bone turnover, and by stimulating the conversion of 25-hydroxyvitamin D (25(OH)D) to the active 1,25-dihydroxyvitamin D (1,25(OH)$_2$D). It decreases serum phosphorus by inhibiting its reabsorption in the proximal tubule of the kidney. The complications of hyperparathyroidism may include kidney stones, renal insufficiency, and osteoporosis. 25(OH)D is the principal circulating vitamin D metabolite. It is converted to 1,25(OH)$_2$D, the biologically active vitamin D metabolite, in the kidney. 1,25(OH)$_2$D increases the intestinal absorption of calcium and phosphorus and regulates skeletal homeostasis by increasing osteoclastic and osteoblastic differentiation. Therefore, a primary increase in vitamin D metabolites would result in an excess of both calcium and phosphorus. Calcitonin decreases serum calcium and phosphorus levels primarily by inhibiting osteoclastic bone resorption. Elevated T$_4$ levels, as seen in hyperthyroidism, occasionally result in hypercalcemia (but not hypophosphatemia) through the stimulation of bone resorption.

41. **(D)** PE: Increased or decreased filling pressure, decreased cardiac output, increased

SVR. Hypovolemic shock: Decreased filling pressure, increased or decreased CO, increased SVR. Septic shock: Decreased filling pressure, increased CO, decreased SVR.

42. **(B)** Vitamin K deficiency would obviously affect those coagulation proteins that are dependent on vitamin K for their function, which includes factors II, VII, IX, and X. Factor V is not dependent on vitamin K for its efficacy.

43. **(B)** The most common cause of constipation in an elderly patient is narcotic analgesics. Barbiturates are not commonly used and do not frequently result in constipation. Neither H_2 receptor antagonists nor PPIs have been implicated in the development of constipation.

44. **(C)** Patients are generally older, with possibly vascular thrombotic episodes, elevated platelets, and a high hematocrit. These patients usually have a normal to low erythropoietin level as opposed to those with a secondary polycythemia in which the level is high.

45. **(A)** A positive secretin test is defined as an elevation in the serum gastrin level by at least 200 pg/mL and is the most sensitive test available for the diagnosis of Zollinger-Ellison syndrome. Carcinoid syndrome is diagnosed by an elevation in the 24-hour excretion of 5-HIAA. Although Zollinger-Ellison syndrome accounts for about 1% of the incidence of peptic ulcer disease, a secretin test is generally not indicated for this disorder unless the diagnosis is suggestive of Zollinger-Ellison syndrome.

46. **(D)** This is another example of a fixed upper airway obstruction. Significant goiters compressing the trachea are not compliant, and the airway narrowing caused by the goiter is not likely to change with changes in the pressure gradient caused by forced inspiratory or expiratory maneuvers. Similarly, tracheal stenosis or fixed tumors that encase the whole trachea may also cause a fixed upper airway obstruction. This will be reflected by a truncation of both the inspiratory and expiratory phases of the flow-volume curve.

47. **(B)** In Lyme disease, the spirochete is inoculated from an infected tick, resulting in a skin lesion called erythema migrans.

48. **(A)** Diabetes insipidus caused by decrease in the secretion of ADH is a common acute complication of pituitary surgery. Findings include increased urination and increased thirst. The urine is very dilute with a low urine osmolality, and the serum sodium level and serum osmolality are often elevated. The opposite findings occur in SIADH, which is associated with hyponatremia, a low serum osmolality, and a high urine osmolality. Diabetes mellitus and hyperthyroidism can cause polyuria and polydipsia but are not complications of pituitary surgery.

49. **(B)** 21α-hydroxylase is the most common cause of CAH, followed by the other enzyme deficiencies.

50. **(B)** When isolates have shown resistance to beta-lactam antibiotics, they may not respond to ceftriaxone alone and vancomycin needs to be added. Acyclovir is useful only in viral or aseptic meningitis, and ampicillin will cover *Listeria* and group B streptococcus, but may not be effective against *Neisseria meningitidis*, which can have a high mortality if untreated.

Practice Test 11
Questions

DIRECTIONS (Questions 1 through 50): Each of the numbered items or incomplete statements in this section is followed by answers or by completions of the statement. Select the ONE lettered answer or completion that is BEST in each case.

1. A deficiency of the red cell membrane component spectrin causes

    (A) hereditary spherocytosis
    (B) pernicious anemia
    (C) Blackfan-Diamond syndrome
    (D) sickle cell anemia
    (E) thalassemia major

2. The most reliable test for detecting a ruptured cervical disk is

    (A) anteroposterior (AP), lateral, and oblique views of the lumbar spine
    (B) technetium bone scan
    (C) cervical myelogram with reformatted computed tomography (CT)
    (D) ultrasound
    (E) magnetic resonance imaging (MRI)

3. If a patient has the most common cause of congenital adrenal hyperplasia (CAH), which of the following levels will be elevated?

    (A) 11-deoxycortisol
    (B) 11-deoxycorticosterone
    (C) aldosterone
    (D) 17-hydroxyprogesterone
    (E) cortisol

4. Which of the following is true concerning sickle cell anemia in adults?

    (A) It is accompanied by iron deficiency.
    (B) It protects against malaria.
    (C) It occurs in 20% of African-Americans in the United States.
    (D) It results from decreased hemoglobin synthesis.
    (E) It produces splenomegaly.

5. Which of the following is a risk factor for the development of osteoporosis?

    (A) excessive alcohol intake
    (B) low-fiber diet
    (C) late menopause
    (D) a good diet
    (E) weight-bearing exercise

6. A 34-year-old woman is diagnosed with a 3-cm left adrenal pheochromocytoma. She read on the Internet that some pheochromocytomas could be familial. Which of the following has a familial association of pheochromocytoma?

    (A) multiple endocrine neoplasia type 1 (MEN 1)
    (B) polyglandular autoimmune syndrome
    (C) Schmidt syndrome
    (D) neurofibromatosis
    (E) hypothyroidism

7. A patient known to have a pheochromocytoma in scheduled for surgery in 2 weeks. What is the most important drug to give her now and for the next 2 weeks in order to prevent serious perioperative complications?

   (A) beta blocker
   (B) alpha blocker
   (C) calcium channel blocker
   (D) diuretic
   (E) angiotensin-converting enzyme (ACE) inhibitor

8. Which of the following conditions does not increase the risk for the development of hepatocellular carcinoma (HCC)?

   (A) hepatitis B and C
   (B) idiopathic hemochromatosis
   (C) alcohol-related cirrhosis
   (D) primary biliary cirrhosis
   (E) vitamin C 1,000 mg/day

9. Which of the following is a class I major histocompatability antigen?

   (A) human lymphocyte antigen (HLA)-A
   (B) HLA-D
   (C) HLA-DR
   (D) HLA-DP
   (E) HLA-DQ

10. What is the most frequent cause of death in women?

   (A) breast cancer
   (B) accidents
   (C) heart attacks
   (D) diabetes
   (E) stroke

11. Regarding neural regulation of the cardiac system, which of the following is correct?

   (A) With positional changes, there is compensatory vasodilation in the venous system.
   (B) Autonomic reflexes are activated through activation of baroreceptors in the aortic arch and carotid bodies.
   (C) Parasympathetic activation results in enhanced myocardial contractility.

   (D) Drugs used to enhance the autonomic reflex mechanism and treat orthostasis include ganglionic blocking drugs.
   (E) The neural system does not affect the heart.

12. A 24-year-old woman presents with galactorrhea and amenorrhea. A prolactin level is 450 ng/mL (normal: 0–19). A pituitary MRI shows a 2.5-cm adenoma. How would you treat her?

   (A) surgery
   (B) radiation
   (C) bromocriptine
   (D) diuretics
   (E) methotrexate

13. A 60-year-old man has preoperative labs and is found to have a hematocrit of 67% and a red cell mass that is elevated. Which further tests would be helpful in confirming the diagnosis?

   (A) platelet count and liver/spleen scan
   (B) chest x-ray
   (C) stress test
   (D) serum folate level
   (E) lung scan

14. A 54-year-old man presents with macrognathia, enlargement of the hands and feet, excessive sweating, sleep apnea, and hypertension. You suspect acromegaly. What is the best screening test?

   (A) random growth hormone (GH) levels
   (B) insulin-like growth factor-1 (IGF-1) levels
   (C) MRI of the pituitary
   (D) IGF-2
   (E) CT of the head

15. Which of the following is a hereditary demyelinating neuropathy without cutaneous manifestation?

   (A) Charcot-Marie-Tooth disease
   (B) neurofibromatosis
   (C) tuberous sclerosis
   (D) Sturge-Weber
   (E) ataxia–telangiectasia

16. A 56-year-old man forms recurrent calcium-based renal calculi. A 24-hour urine collection reveals elevated levels of calcium excretion. Which class of diuretic can be used therapeutically for its hypocalciuric effects?

(A) carbonic anhydrase inhibitors
(B) loop diuretics
(C) thiazide diuretics
(D) potassium-sparing diuretics
(E) all diuretics

17. Which of the following is the most frequent complication following total hip arthroplasty?

(A) infection
(B) deep venous thrombosis (DVT)
(C) anterior dislocation
(D) posterior dislocation
(E) unrecognized nickel allergy

18. Patients at highest risk for heart attack include those with

(A) high levels of lipoprotein a [Lp(a)]
(B) low levels of Lp(a)
(C) a family history of heart attack before the age of 70
(D) heavily calcified coronary arteries
(E) highly elevated HDL levels

19. A 74-year-old man with small cell carcinoma of the lungs is hospitalized with lethargy, nausea, and vomiting. His serum Na is 126 mEq/L, and urinary spot sodium is greater than 1%. His most likely diagnosis is

(A) primary polydipsia
(B) renal failure
(C) congestive heart failure (CHF)
(D) syndrome of inappropriate antidiuretic hormone secretion (SIADH)
(E) factitious hyponatremia

20. Following a transurethral resection of the prostate (TURP), a patient with congestive heart failure (CHF) is noted to have crackles on lung exam and bilateral lower extremity edema. He is somewhat confused and nause-

ated. His serum Na is 129 mEq/L and spot urinary sodium is less than 1%. Management should include

(A) a 500-cc bolus of normal saline
(B) albuterol nebulizer treatments
(C) lorazepam 1 mg IV
(D) administration of a diuretic
(E) rapid saline infusion

21. Plaque formation is caused by

(A) calcification in the wall of the blood vessel
(B) disruption of the epithelium by deposits of cholesterol
(C) deposits of low-density lipoprotein (LDL) and other fatty materials in the vessel endothelium
(D) invasion of intact vessel walls by white blood cells
(E) platelets adhering to epithelial cells, which are damaged by fatty materials

Refer to Figure 11.1 for question 22.

22. Culture of the green-colored nails shown in Figure 11.1 is most likely to grow which organism?

(A) *Klebsiella pneumoniae*
(B) *Staphylococcus aureus*
(C) *Pseudomonas aeruginosa*
(D) *Serratia marcescens*
(E) *Clostridium perfringens*

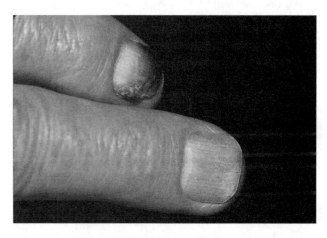

Figure 11.1

23. Which of the following is the most likely etiology of vitiligo?

   (A) autoimmune
   (B) drug-induced
   (C) infectious
   (D) neoplastic
   (E) traumatic

24. For the week prior to presentation, a 57-year-old man has had an acute febrile illness with coughing, rigors, and production of purulent sputum. A chest x-ray reveals an area of consolidation in the right upper lobe and his white blood counts are elevated. He is admitted to the hospital and intravenous antibiotics are started. Sputum cultures return with mixed oral flora, and blood cultures are without growth. Despite a third-generation cephalosporin, in addition to a macrolide, the patient continues to spike fevers with a persistent leukocytosis. Which of the following should have been adequately treated by the medication given?

   (A) mycoplasma pneumonia
   (B) development of an empyema
   (C) penicillin-resistant organism
   (D) development of an abscess
   (E) postobstructive pneumonia
   (F) malignancy

25. The Bentiromide test would be useful in the diagnosis of which of the following disorders?

   (A) Zollinger-Ellison syndrome
   (B) pancreatic insufficiency
   (C) acute pancreatitis
   (D) biliary pancreatitis
   (E) hepatitis

26. Absorption of vitamin B_{12} would be impaired in which of the following conditions?

   (A) gastroesophageal reflux disease (GERD)
   (B) peptic ulcer
   (C) excessive caffeine intake
   (D) pancreatic insufficiency or ileal resection
   (E) *Helicobacter pylori* infection

27. Histamine-2 (H_2) receptor antagonists specifically block the H_2 receptor on which cell in the stomach?

   (A) parietal
   (B) mucous neck gland
   (C) enterochromaffin-like (ECL)
   (D) chief
   (E) stromal

28. Which cell in the stomach is responsible for the synthesis and release of pepsinogen following meal stimulation?

   (A) parietal
   (B) ECL
   (C) chief
   (D) mucous neck gland
   (E) stromal

29. A 52-year-old man has developed fasting hyperglycemia. On careful history, he also reports difficulties with arthralgias, weakness, and impotence. Examination reveals a diffuse bronze hyperpigmentation of his skin. Blood work is significant for moderate elevations in his transaminases, and a chest x-ray reveals a mildly enlarged cardiac shadow. What test is most likely to suggest the cause of this patient's symptoms?

   (A) glycosylated hemoglobin
   (B) fat aspirate with Congo red staining
   (C) transferrin saturation
   (D) morning cortisol level
   (E) antinuclear antibody (ANA) and sedimentation rate

30. Which immunoglobulin (Ig) is most involved in anaphylactic reactions?

   (A) IgA
   (B) IgG
   (C) IgD
   (D) IgE
   (E) IgM

31. A 45-year-old woman is diagnosed with nephrogenic diabetes insipidus. Which of the following can make her condition worse?

(A) hypocalcemia

(B) hypoglycemia

(C) hyponatremia

(D) hypokalemia

(E) hypoalbuminemia

Questions 32 and 33

A 16-year-old girl is found to have a 2-cm nodule in her right thyroid lobe on routine examination. Her family history is significant for a mother and a younger sister with medullary thyroid cancer (MTC). Her mother also has primary hyperparathyroidism. A fine-needle aspirate reveals findings consistent with MTC.

32. Which of the following genes is affected?

(A) MENIN

(B) VHL

(C) Merlin

(D) RET

(E) FAP

33. The patient undergoes a total thyroidectomy without complication. Which of the following hormone levels will be useful to assess disease recurrence in this patient's follow-up?

(A) thyroglobulin

(B) thyroid-stimulating hormone (TSH)

(C) antithyroid peroxidase antibodies

(D) calcitonin

(E) CA 19-9

34. What is the mode of *Ehrlichia* transmission?

(A) dog tick (*Dermacentor variabilis*) or wood tick (*Dermacentor andersoni*)

(B) deer tick (*Ixodes scapularis*)

(C) *Borrelia burgdorferi*

(D) *Treponema pallidum*

(E) *Rickettsia rickettsii*

Questions 35 and 36

35. In what percentage of first-trimester spontaneous abortions are chromosomal abnormalities found?

(A) 10%

(B) 20%

(C) 50%

(D) 90%

(E) 100%

36. Of the chromosomal abnormalities found in analysis of fetal tissue from first-trimester spontaneous abortions, what is the most common specific anomaly?

(A) Down syndrome (trisomy 21)

(B) trisomy 13

(C) Turner's syndrome (45,X)

(D) trisomy 18

(E) osteogenica

37. The presence of hemolysis is indicated by which of the following?

(A) increased red blood cell survival

(B) absent or reduced serum haptoglobin

(C) a decreased number of reticulocytes

(D) decreased serum lactate dehydrogenase (LDH)

(E) microcytic red blood cell indices

38. The earliest sign of impending uncal herniation due to increased intracranial pressure may be

(A) pupillary meiosis

(B) pupillary mydriasis

(C) hemiparesis

(D) loss of oculocephalic reflex ("doll's-eye")

(E) loss of oculovestibular reflex (cold-water calorics)

39. A 70-year-old white man presents with pain in his right groin of 6 months' duration, lytic and blastic lesions on pelvic x-ray, arthritic changes in the right hip, an elevated serum alkaline phosphatase, and increased urinary pyridium cross-links on assay. What is the most likely diagnosis?

(A) metastatic carcinoma of the prostate

(B) chondrosarcoma of the pelvis

(C) multiple myeloma

(D) Paget's disease

(E) fracture

40. A known cancer patient presents with spastic paraparesis, urinary retention, loss of distal leg sensation, and vertebral spine pain. What do the clinical signs indicate?

    (A) stroke
    (B) B_6 toxicity
    (C) pernicious anemia
    (D) trauma
    (E) possible spinal cord compression

41. Of the following primary neoplasms, the one most likely to metastasize to the brain is

    (A) osteosarcoma
    (B) squamous cell
    (C) basal cell
    (D) prostate
    (E) renal cell

42. An 85-year-old woman complains of urinary urgency and frequency and dysuria on a routine visit to her primary care physician. A urinanalysis is positive for nitrite and leukocytes. Microscopic analysis reveals rod-shaped organisms. Which of the following is the most likely organism?

    (A) *Enterococcus faecalis*
    (B) *Klebsiella*
    (C) *Proteus*
    (D) *Pseudomonas*
    (E) *Escherichia coli*

Questions 43 and 44

A 57-year-old woman is being treated for type 2 diabetes, hypertension, and dyslipidemia. Her medications include repaglinide, metformin, pioglitazone, quinapril, and atorvastatin. During a follow-up visit, she complains of an annoying cough.

43. Which of the following medication substitutions is most likely to relieve her symptoms?

    (A) atorvastatin → niacin
    (B) pioglitazone → rosiglitazone
    (C) metformin → phenformin
    (D) repaglinide → chlorpropamide
    (E) quinapril → losartan

44. The patient is admitted to the hospital with severe dyspnea at rest and is found to have hypoxia and bilateral pulmonary edema. An echocardiogram reveals poor systolic function with an estimated ejection fraction of 20%. Which of the following two medications should be discontinued in this patient?

    (A) pioglitazone and metformin
    (B) glipizide and pioglitazone
    (C) quinapril and metformin
    (D) atorvastatin and quinapril
    (E) glipizide and atorvastatin

45. Bladder cancer in the United States has which of the following characteristics?

    (A) transitional cell histology in 90% of cases
    (B) painful hematuria
    (C) low rate of local recurrence
    (D) aniline dyes as an occupational exposure proven to have no effect
    (E) higher incidence in women than in men

46. What is the most common benign mesenchymal tumor of the stomach?

    (A) lipoma
    (B) schwannoma
    (C) leiomyoma
    (D) glomus tumor
    (E) adenoma

47. What is the primary predisposing factor for actinic keratosis?

    (A) inheritance
    (B) chemical exposure
    (C) cigarette smoking
    (D) sunlight exposure
    (E) autoimmune disease

48. A 66-year-old man initially presents with a large pleural effusion. A thoracentesis is performed showing malignant cells. What is the most likely primary cancer?

    (A) colon cancer
    (B) lung cancer
    (C) pancreatic cancer

(D) lymphoma

(E) mesothelioma

49. Which of the following is the most important histopathologic indicator of the prognosis of stage 1 malignant melanoma?

(A) thickness of tumor

(B) density of host inflammatory response

(C) mitotic index

(D) ulceration

(E) radial extent of tumor

50. Following primary infection with human immunodeficiency virus (HIV), initial viremia is maximal at

(A) 3 to 4 days

(B) 1 to 3 weeks

(C) 3 to 6 weeks

(D) 3 to 6 months

(E) 6 to 12 months

Answers and Explanations

1. **(A)** Hereditary spherocytosis is a red cell membrane defect. There is a genetically determined abnormality in the membrane polypeptide spectrin. The degree of deficiency correlates with the degree of spherocytosis. Pernicious anemia is caused by low B_{12} or folate. Sickle cell anemia has a single amino acid substitution in the beta chain of hemoglobin, and thalassemia is caused by decreased production of the beta chain. Aplastic anemia is associated with Blackfan-Diamond syndrome.

2. **(C)** Technetium bone scanning shows areas of increased bone turnover and is very reliable for detecting fractures not visible on plain x-rays, such as early stress fractures and bone tumors, both primary and metastatic, that cause reactive bone formation. MRI scanning is reliable in detecting a ruptured cervical disk but cannot be used on a patient with a pacemaker. The "gold standard" for detecting a ruptured cervical disk is a myelogram with postmyelogram reformatted CT scan.

3. **(D)** In 21α-hydroxylase deficiency, 17-hydroxyprogesterone will be high.

4. **(B)** Sickle cell anemia patients in areas with endemic malaria do better since this is an evolutionary response to malaria. Since the hemolyzed cell products release iron, there is excess, rather than deficient, iron. Only 1% of African-Americans have full-blown sickle cell anemia, but 10% or more have sickle trait. The spleen is generally autoinfarcted and thus small. Anemia results from production of abnormal hemoglobin and the subsequent hemolysis of the red blood cells containing the hemoglobin; it is not the result of decreased hemoglobin synthesis.

5. **(A)** Alcohol interferes with Ca^{++} absorption. Dietary fiber interferes with vitamin D absorption. Estrogen stimulates osteoblast function.

6. **(D)** Pheochromocytoma is associated with neurofibromatosis and MEN 2A and 2B (not MEN 1). Schmidt syndrome is the combination of adrenal insufficiency and Hashimoto's thyroiditis.

7. **(B)** An alpha blocker, such as phenoxybenzamine, is given for 2 weeks preoperatively. A beta blocker may be added at some point if tachycardia develops, but it should not be given prior to alpha blockade because unopposed alpha receptor activation may result in worsening hypertension.

8. **(D)** HCC is by far the most common primary malignancy of the liver. The most important etiologic factors appear to be hepatitis B and C. Alcohol-related cirrhosis is a frequent cause, although in many there is concurrent hepatitis B or C. Hemochromatosis in its cirrhotic stage is associated with the development of HCC in 10% to 15% of cases. Primary biliary cirrhosis, primary sclerosing cholangitis, Wilson's disease, and autoimmune cirrhosis rarely develop into HCC.

9. **(A)** HLA-A, -B and -C are class I antigens that consist of one heavy glycopeptide chain noncovalently linked with a short microglob-

ulin chain. The other answers are class II MHC antigens.

10. **(C)**   Heart disease and heart attacks are the number one killers of women in America and other developed countries throughout the world. Cardiovascular disease kills over 500,000 women in the United States annually. It claims more women's lives than breast cancer, accidents, and diabetes combined.

11. **(B)**   Positional changes result in a variety of compensatory changes that facilitate maintenance of normal blood pressure in the upright position. These include enhanced vasomotor tone, which results primarily through sympathetic activation. Sympathetic activation enhances myocardial function. Drugs such as ganglionic blocking drugs can impair the autonomic reflex mechanism and result in or worsen orthostasis.

12. **(C)**   Prolactinomas, no matter what size they are, are treated medically. Dopamine agonists (such as bromocriptine and cabergoline) shrink the adenoma and lower prolactin. Surgery and radiation are reserved for patients who cannot tolerate medical treatment.

13. **(A)**   An absolute erythrocytosis was detected by red cell mass, and thus polycythemia vera, either primary or secondary, needs to be evaluated for. Thus, the usual tests include arterial blood gas that is normal; splenomegaly by scan; elevated B_{12}; elevated platelets and leukocyte levels, since this is a myeloproliferative disorder; and an elevated alkaline phosphatase level. Although a secondary polycythemia may be evident from lung disease, a lung scan would not be useful as initial testing.

14. **(B)**   IGF-1 is the best screening test for acromegaly. There is an overlap in GH levels between normal and acromegalic people. MRI is done after the diagnosis is confirmed. IGF-2 is not increased in acromegaly.

15. **(A)**   Charcot-Marie-Tooth disease is a hereditary demyelinating neuropathy associated with pes cavus foot deformity but not with skin changes. All of the other options are phakomatoses and include skin manifestations such as adenoma sebaceum and a hypopigmented leaf-shaped macule (tuberous sclerosis), café au lait spots (neurofibromatosis), facial angioma (Sturge-Weber), and telangiectasias (ataxia–telangiectasia).

16. **(C)**   Unlike loop diuretics, thiazide diuretics inhibit NaCl reabsorption at the cortical diluting segment. Furthermore, they do not inhibit calcium reabsorption like loop diuretics, which causes an increase in calcium excretion; instead, they have a hypocalciuric effect both acutely and during chronic administration.

17. **(B)**   DVT occurs in almost 50% of patients undergoing total hip arthroplasty when some form of DVT prophylaxis is not used. Most of these clots are asymptomatic. Dislocation occurs in less than 4% and is related to the position of the components and surgical approach used (anterior or posterior). The deep infection rate following total hip arthroplasty is less than 1%.

18. **(A)**   High levels of a certain type of lipoprotein a in the blood are associated with an increased risk of heart attack. Over a 10-year period, patients with highest levels of Lp(a) are 70% more likely to have a heart attack than patients with the lowest levels of Lp(a). Patients whose parents had a heart attack before age 60 are at higher risk for developing coronary artery disease (CAD) at a young age. Patients with CAD whose arteries have a great deal of fatty plaque may be at higher risk of heart attack than patients with calcification. Fatty plaque is more dangerous because it is more likely to rupture.

19. **(D)**   Characteristic features of SIADH include hyponatremia with excretion of urine that is not maximally dilute. Disorders associated with SIADH include malignancies, pulmonary diseases, and central nervous system (CNS) disorders. It most commonly occurs with bronchogenic carcinomas.

20. **(D)** This patient is at risk for volume overload with his CHF. Certain procedures such as a TURP are particularly notable for marked volume expansion caused by absorption of large amounts of osmotically active irrigant used in the case. The patient clearly has a dilutional hyponatremia, and part of the management involves encouraging a diuresis of excess fluid.

21. **(C)** LDL cholesterol produces toxins that damage endothelial cells of the inside wall of the artery. This damage contributes to the formation of tiny endothelial lesions. Other fatty materials in the bloodstream (e.g., triglycerides) are attracted to the lesions and begin to build up there. White blood cells are attracted to the site of damage and cause the lining of the artery to become "sticky," resulting in deposition of even more LDL molecules. Platelets collect over the site, release more irritating substances, and trap more fatty particles and white blood cells. This gradual buildup of fatty materials and toxins is known as plaque.

22. **(C)** Green discoloration of the nail is most suggestive of *Pseudomonas* infection.

23. **(A)** Autoimmune mechanism with an underlying genetic predisposition is the most likely cause of vitiligo.

24. **(A)** The patient's clinical presentation is consistent with an acute pneumonia. Response to empiric antimicrobial therapy should be seen within 48 to 72 hours. In the nonresponding patient, several important considerations must be made, including whether the diagnosis and likely pathogens involved are correct. Penicillin-resistant *Streptococcus pneumoniae* is increasing in incidence and should be considered in certain populations. Penicillin resistance is often accompanied by resistance to other antibiotics, including macrolides, and therefore the "double coverage" of *Streptococcus* with the additional macrolide is not necessarily reassurance that a resistant species is responsible for the poor clinical response. Unusual or-

ganisms must also be considered, such as viral, fungal, and mycobacterial pathogens. Mycoplasma pneumonia is considered an "atypical pneumonia" but should have been well covered by the patient's macrolide, and are notably covered by most recommended empiric regimens for community acquired pneumonia. If the diagnosis is correct, then complicating factors should be sought in the nonresponsive patient such as the development of a pulmonary abscess or an empyema. Although sometimes difficult to tease out in the acute illness, postobstructive pneumonia should also be considered in those at risk for the development of a malignancy. Primary malignancies may also mimic a pneumonia such as may occur with bronchoalveolar cell carcinoma.

25. **(B)** The Bentiromide test is a noninvasive test of pancreatic function. It relies on the presence of a normal amount of duodenal chemotrypsin, which is necessary to cleave free para-aminobenzoic acid (PABA). If sufficient quantities of the enzyme are present, it implies normal pancreatic function, resulting in the release of free PABA, which is ultimately excreted into the urine.

26. **(D)** *H. pylori,* GERD, peptic ulcer, and caffeine have not been associated with the development of vitamin B_{12} deficiency. B_{12} absorption will be affected in celiac disease and pernicious anemia.

27. **(A)** The H_2 receptor is present on the basolateral surface of the parietal cell and is responsible for the stimulation of the H^+,K^+ ATPase acid pump. The H_2 receptor is not present on either of the other cell types listed.

28. **(C)** The chief cell is localized to the base of the gastric gland and is responsible for the synthesis and release of pepsinogen following meal stimulation. The parietal cell is the acid-producing cell of the stomach and lines the gastric gland. The ECL cell of the stomach is the histamine-containing cell of the stomach and releases histamine in response to meal stimulation. The histamine in turn stim-

ulates the parietal cell to release acid through the H_2 receptor.

29. **(C)** The patient has evidence of multiorgan dysfunction: endocrine, cardiac, skin, liver, joints, and pancreas. The characteristic combination of diabetes and hyperpigmentation (bronze diabetes) in the setting of abnormal liver tests suggest the possibility of hemochromatosis. Hemochromatosis is a state of iron overload, and deposition into any organ system can cause dysfunction over time. This includes diabetes, heart failure, secondary hypogonadism, cirrhosis, and hypothyroidism. Recently, mutations in HFE gene have been found to be associated with hereditary hemochromatosis; however, genetic testing is generally not the first-line diagnostic test for an index case. The most appropriate screening test is probably transferrin saturation, which will be elevated in patients with hemochromatosis. Glycosylated hemoglobin will give an idea of the control of the patient's diabetes but is otherwise not helpful in the diagnosis. The fat aspirate may suggest amyloidosis, which is also a multiorgan process but has different manifestations that may include peripheral neuropathy, easy bruisability, heart failure, neuropathy, and macroglossia. Morning cortisol level would help diagnose adrenal insufficiency, and although Addison's disease may cause hyperpigmentation and some of the constitutional symptoms, the other findings would not be characteristic of adrenal insufficiency.

30. **(D)** IgE is a reagenic antibody involved in anaphylactic reactions.

31. **(D)** Hypokalemia and hypercalcemia can cause nephrogenic diabetes insipidus.

32. **(D)** MTC is sporadic in 80% of cases and familial in 20%. Familial MTC can occur in isolation or in association with multiple endocrine neoplasia (MEN) syndrome 2A or 2B. MEN 2A consists of the triad of MTC, primary hyperparathyroidism, and pheochromocytoma. MEN 2B is characterized by multiple mucosal neuromas, MTC, and pheo-

chromocytoma. All of the familial MTC syndromes involve an activating mutation in the RET proto-oncogene. MEN 1, which is characterized by pituitary tumors, primary hyperparathyroidism, and pancreatic tumors, is caused by a mutation in the MENIN gene. VHL gene mutations are associated with von Hippel–Lindau disease, Merlin mutations with type 2 neurofibromatosis, and FAP mutations with familial polyposis coli.

33. **(D)** MTC is caused by a neoplastic process in the parafollicular C-cells of the thyroid gland. These cells produce calcitonin, which can be used as a tumor marker in these patients. Because C-cells do not produce thyroglobulin, this protein is not a useful tumor marker for MTC. The TSH is elevated in patients who have had their thyroid gland removed but is useful only in the assessment of thyroid hormone replacement dosing and does not give any information regarding recurrence of MTC. CA 19-9 may be elevated in cancers of gastrointestinal origin. Antithyroid peroxidase antibodies are used to help in the diagnosis of benign autoimmune thyroid disease.

34. **(B)** *Babesia* and *Ehrlichia* can both be carried by the *Ixodes* tick. This is the same tick that carries *Borrelia burgdorferi*, the spirochete that is the cause of Lyme disease.

35–36. **(35-C, 36-C)** At least half of the time that chromosomal analysis is made of fetal tissue from spontaneous abortions, chromosomal abnormalities are found. Taken as a group, autosomal trisomies are the most frequent anomaly, of which trisomy 13, 16, 18, 21, and 26 are the most common and account for about 50% of anomalies found. After this, 45,X or Turner's syndrome is the next most common and therefore the single most common anomaly.

37. **(B)** In an attempt to compensate for a shortened survival in the hemolysis setting, the bone marrow increases reticulocyte production. Haptoglobin is consumed in the process of binding the excess free hemoglobin during

red cell destruction. LDH is present in increased amounts, again due to increased release from the destroyed red cell. Red cell indices are usually normal and are therefore not useful in detecting hemolysis.

38. **(B)** Pupillary meiosis (constriction) may be seen in structural pontine lesions. The other findings may appear later in the course of brain stem herniation. The third cranial nerve is most peripheral at the midbrain, and the pupillary fascicles are most peripheral within this nerve. Therefore, pupillary dilatation is often the earliest sign of impending brain herniation.

39. **(D)** Active Paget's disease is characterized by a high rate of bone turnover producing elevated serum alkaline phosphatase and type I collagen breakdown products (pyridinium cross-links). Serum acid phosphatase level is elevated with metastatic carcinoma of the prostate. Monoclonal Bence Jones protein detectable in the urine is common with multiple myeloma.

40. **(E)** Any of the clinical sign listed may be associated with impending spinal cord compression. Prominent spine pain may suggest a metastatic etiology of the myelopathy.

41. **(E)** While prostate cancer commonly spreads to bone and can metastasize to the skull or vertebral spine, it typically does not involve brain parenchyma. Common metastatic brain tumors include lung, breast, and skin (melanoma).

42. **(E)** *E. coli* is the most common cause of urinary tract infections, accounting for 85% of community-acquired and 50% of hospital-acquired infections.

43. **(E)** Chronic cough is one of the most common side effects of therapy with an angiotensin-converting enzyme (ACE) inhibitor. ACE is a kininase, and ACE inhibitors may lead to an increase in bradykinin levels, which may lead to cough. Angiotensin II blockers such as losartan do not affect this pathway and therefore can be substituted when a patient does not tolerate an ACE inhibitor due to cough. Cough is not a common side effect of any of the other therapies listed.

44. **(A)** Pioglitazone may cause excessive fluid retention and therefore should not be used in New York Heart Association class III or IV congestive heart failure. Metformin is contraindicated in any patient who may be predisposed to the development of lactic acidosis, such as in patients with significant liver or kidney dysfunction, sepsis, severe CHF, or other severe illness. Quinapril is an ACE inhibitor and is indicated in the treatment of heart failure. Atorvastatin is not contraindicated in this condition. Repaglinide may be continued if necessary to control her blood glucose levels.

45. **(A)** Ninety percent of bladder cancers in the United States are of transitional cell origin. Schistosomiasis is a known cause of squamous cell carcinoma, particularly in endemic areas such as the Middle East. There is a known association with aniline dye exposure, and men are more frequently affected than women. Patients with bladder tumors generally present with painless hematuria or signs of bladder infection or irritability. In early stages, surgery may be effective, but they tend to recur locally and thus need aggressive follow-up and observation.

46. **(C)** Leiomyoma, a smooth-muscle tumor, is the most common benign tumor of the stomach. Leiomyosarcomas can occur, and thus large stromal-appearing tumors need to be evaluated for this as well. Adenomas are of epithelial origin, and the other tumor types are not common to the stomach.

47. **(D)** Actinic keratosis is due to prolonged exposure to the actinic rays of the sun. The lesions are usually found on areas such as the face, hands, and any other surface chronically exposed to sun. Although these lesions are not malignant, they can lead to either squamous or basal cell skin cancers. Treatment is wide surgical excision.

48. **(B)** Most pleural effusions are caused by malignant disease and generally those with adenocarcinomas. The usual sites are lung in men and breast in women. Colon and pancreas can cause effusions but not usually on presentation.

49. **(A)** Depth of invasion is the most important prognostic indicator for stage 1 malignant melanoma.

50. **(C)** The majority of patients infected with HIV experience an acute syndrome approximately 3 to 6 weeks following primary infection; features include fever, lymphadenopathy, headache, arthralgias/myalgias, lethargy/malaise, and erythematous maculopapular rash.

Practice Test 12
Questions

DIRECTIONS (Questions 1 through 50): Each of the numbered items or incomplete statements in this section is followed by answers or by completions of the statement. Select the ONE lettered answer or completion that is BEST in each case.

1. An 18-year-old woman comes to your office to discuss birth control methods since she is considering initiation of sexual activity with her current boyfriend. Which of the following methods, assuming proper and consistent use, is the most effective at preventing pregnancy?

   (A) combination oral contraceptives (OCs)
   (B) diaphragm and spermicide
   (C) intrauterine device (IUD)
   (D) condoms
   (E) rhythm

2. A 17-year-old girl presents with severe fatigue, anorexia, and weight loss. Addison's disease (primary adrenal insufficiency) is suspected. Which of the following is usually present in autoimmune primary adrenal insufficiency?

   (A) elevated aldosterone levels
   (B) hyperpigmentation
   (C) exaggerated response of cortisol to a cosyntropin (synthetic adrenocorticotropic hormone [ACTH]) injection
   (D) decreased ACTH levels
   (E) elevated chondroitin

3. Patients presenting with *Helicobacter pylori* infection may develop

   (A) reflux esophagitis
   (B) peptic ulcer disease
   (C) celiac sprue
   (D) colon cancer
   (E) colonic polyps

4. A 69-year-old man from Egypt is seen in your clinic for gross hematuria. A detailed history reveals a history of schistosomiasis. Cystoscopy reveals a suspicious bladder lesion, which is subsequently biopsied. The most common tumor given this history is

   (A) small cell carcinoma
   (B) renal cell carcinoma
   (C) pheochromocytoma
   (D) squamous cell carcinoma
   (E) transitional cell carcinoma

5. Which is the most dangerous and unwise test to perform in evaluating the patient with a suspected dissecting aortic aneurysm?

   (A) electrocardiogram (ECG)
   (B) echocardiogram
   (C) magnetic resonance imaging (MRI)
   (D) computed tomography (CT)
   (E) exercise stress test

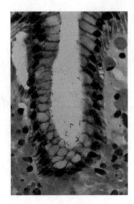

Figure 12.1

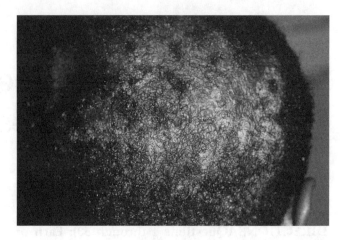

Figure 12.2

6. Figure 12.1 demonstrates which of the following organisms?

   (A) *H. pylori*
   (B) *Shigella* sp.
   (C) *Escherichia coli*
   (D) *Clostridium difficile*
   (E) *Staphylococcus aureus*

7. A 56-year-old man is diagnosed with SIADH (syndrome of inappropriate antidiuretic hormone secretion). Which of the following combinations of tests is consistent with the diagnosis?

	Plasma Osmolality	Urine Osmolality
(A)	Low	Low
(B)	Low	High
(C)	High	High
(D)	High	Low

8. What viral cofactor is currently felt to be a major factor for the development of squamous cell cancer of the cervix?

   (A) herpes simplex virus type 2 (HSV-2)
   (B) human immunodeficiency virus (HIV)
   (C) human papillomavirus (HPV)
   (D) hepatitis B virus
   (E) parvovirus

9. Which of the following markers is associated with colorectal carcinoma?

   (A) alpha-fetoprotein (AFP)
   (B) human chorionic gonadotropin (hCG)
   (C) carcinoembryonic antigen (CEA)

   (D) hypoglycemic factor
   (E) prostate-specific antigen (PSA)

10. What is the most likely causative agent of the scalp rash in this 6-year-old African-American boy (see Figure 12.2)?

    (A) dermatophyte
    (B) yeast
    (C) virus
    (D) bacteria
    (E) louse infestation

11. A 30-year-old woman has been bothered by symptoms consistent with angioedema. The episodes have generally been self-limited and are typically not painful, erythematous, nor pruritic. Recently, she was seen in the emergency department (ED) due to acute dyspnea, and she was admitted to the hospital for treatment and observation. She was suspected to have had a reaction to a food that she ate that day and was treated as if she had anaphylaxis. She also reports having bouts of abdominal pain for most of her life and a separate episode recently also requiring a visit to the ED. The diagnosis of hereditary angioneurotic edema is suspected, and a C1-inhibitor level is ordered, but returns normal. What is the next best appropriate step?

    (A) skin testing for food allergies
    (B) C1-inhibitor functional test
    (C) initiation of chronic antihistamine therapy

(D) bone marrow biopsy to rule out systemic mastocytosis

(E) IgE level

12. Cutaneous vasculitis is an example of which type of immune reaction?

(A) type I

(B) type II

(C) type III

(D) type IV

(E) type V

13. A patient is found to have a serum sodium of 118 mEq/L. If you correct the sodium too quickly, what complication may occur?

(A) cerebral bleeding

(B) pulmonary edema

(C) deep venous thrombosis (DVT)

(D) central pontine myelinolysis

(E) peripheral edema

14. In cases of childhood sexual abuse, approximately what percentage of the time is the assailant known to the child?

(A) 10%

(B) 25%

(C) 50%

(D) 80%

(E) 95%

15. A 27-year-old man with celiac sprue presents with proximal muscle weakness and bone pain. Which of the following serum values are consistent with severe vitamin D deficiency?

	(A)	(B)	(C)	(D)	(E)
Calcium	High	Low	Low	Low	Low
Phosphate	Low	High	Low	High	Normal
Parathyroid hormone (PTH)	Low	Normal	High	Low	Normal
1,25-dihydroxyvitamin D	High	Low	Low	Low	High

16. Malignant melanomas typically

(A) do not metastasize via the lymphatic vessels

(B) do not arise de novo

(C) arise in the papillary dermis

(D) arise in areas protected from the sun

(E) metastasize hematogenously

17. Which of the following is characteristic of a unicameral bone cyst?

(A) It develops a distance from the metaphyseal bone adjacent to the physis.

(B) Uncommon sites are the proximal humerus and proximal femur.

(C) A geographic pattern of bone destruction with cortical thinning and expansion is seen on x-ray.

(D) Multiple aspirations and injections with methylprednisolone rarely result in healing.

(E) It is commonly found at the center of long bones.

18. A 62-year-old diabetic woman presents to the ED with fever, vomiting, and left flank pain. She had recently been treated for an *E. coli* urinary tract infection (UTI). Lab values reveal a white blood cell (WBC) count 26,000. A KUB (kidney, ureter, and bladder exam) reveals a collection of gas in the left upper quadrant. Her likely diagnosis is

(A) gastric distention

(B) small bowel obstruction

(C) hydronephrosis

(D) xanthogranulomatous pyelonephritis

(E) emphysematous pyelonephritis

19. Which of the following tests is unnecessary for a workup following the finding of a moth-eaten lesion in the femoral neck of a 64-year-old white woman?

(A) bone scan

(B) chest CT scan

(C) hip ultrasound

(D) liver–spleen scan

(E) breast exam

20. A 36-year-old G2P1 at 22 weeks of intrauterine pregnancy (IUP) presents to her physician on a routine visit. A urinalysis reveals leukocytes and is nitrite positive. A urine culture is sent and reveals an *E. coli* infection with a significant colony count. She denies having any urinary tract symptoms. Ideal management would be

   (A) to increase hydration
   (B) treatment with a tetracycline
   (C) treatment with a sulfonamide
   (D) treatment with biofeedback
   (E) treatment with a penicillin

21. Which of the following best describes a comminuted fracture?

   (A) a fracture in which the bone penetrates the skin
   (B) a fracture with many fragments at the fracture site
   (C) a fracture communicating with a joint
   (D) a fracture caused by a twisting injury
   (E) a fracture fragment pulled off with a ligament or tendon

22. The release of which of the following substances results in the amplification of glucose-induced insulin release?

   (A) glucagon
   (B) somatostatin
   (C) gastrin
   (D) epinephrine
   (E) norepinephrine

23. Which of the following markers is associated with hydatidiform mole?

   (A) AFP
   (B) hCG
   (C) CEA
   (D) PSA
   (E) CA 121

24. Patients may have multiple contraindications to OC use. For which of the following patients would you prescribe an OC?

   (A) a patient with active liver disease
   (B) a patient with an estrogen-dependent tumor
   (C) a patient with a history of previous thromboemboembolism
   (D) a patient with a prior stroke
   (E) a patient with diabetes

25. A 26-year-old female patient newly diagnosed with porphyria cutanea tarda (PCT) should avoid exposure to which of the following medications?

   (A) isotretinoin
   (B) warfarin
   (C) ibuprofen
   (D) OCs
   (E) penicillin

26. Sickle cell disease can result in

   (A) mesenteric adenitis
   (B) pancreatitis
   (C) osteomyelitis
   (D) diplopia
   (E) pleurisy

27. Which of the following causative agents is a risk factor for the development of angiosarcoma of the liver?

   (A) dietary fat
   (B) cyclamates
   (C) tobacco
   (D) alcohol
   (E) vinyl chloride

28. What is the most common benign breast tumor in premenopausal women?

   (A) lipoma
   (B) hemangioma
   (C) fibroadenoma
   (D) cystic fibroma
   (E) intraductal papilloma

29. A 19-year-old woman presents with the primary complaint of hirsutism, worsening since she entered puberty. She further notes that she has always had very irregular menstrual cycles. Examination reveals an obese young woman with thick, pigmented hair in a male distribution. A pelvic examination is difficult due to her obesity. Which of the following is likely to be true of this patient?

    (A) Serum androgens are likely to be lowered.
    (B) Polycystic ovaries are seen in this disorder.
    (C) There is a decreased likelihood of impaired glucose intolerance or frank type 2 diabetes.
    (D) Menstrual cycles are normal.
    (E) This condition presents late in life.

30. Spontaneous bacterial peritonitis occurring in the setting of ascites is most likely caused by

    (A) *Pseudomonas* sp.
    (B) *E. coli*
    (C) *Salmonella*
    (D) *C. difficile*
    (E) *Staphylococcus*

31. A 43-year-old woman presents with hirsutism, amenorrhea, deepening of the voice, and temporal balding. Her dehydroepiandrosterone sulfate (DHEA-S) level is very high. What is the next step?

    (A) ultrasound of the ovaries
    (B) CT scan of the adrenals
    (C) MRI of the pituitary
    (D) hysterosalpingogram
    (E) serum thyroid function testing

32. Which of the following lipoproteins contains the highest concentration of triglycerides?

    (A) low-density lipoprotein (LDL)
    (B) high-density lipoprotein (HDL)
    (C) intermediate-density lipoprotein (IDL)
    (D) very-low-density lipoprotein (VLDL)
    (E) lipoprotein a [Lp(a)]

33. The blood protein thrombin is known to

    (A) form clots by complexing with fibrin
    (B) require vitamin K in its activated form
    (C) contain gamma-carboxyglutamate residues
    (D) have an enzymatic specificity similar to trypsin
    (E) be an oligomeric protein

34. Urticaria is an example of which type of immune reaction?

    (A) type I
    (B) type II
    (C) type III
    (D) type IV
    (E) type V

35. Korsakoff's syndrome may manifest as

    (A) amnestic syndrome
    (B) global confusion
    (C) ataxia of gait
    (D) horizontal gaze palsy
    (E) nystagmus

36. Atrial fibrillation

    (A) results from rapid spontaneous firing of the sinus node
    (B) can result in embolus
    (C) is related to disease in the atrioventricular (AV) node
    (D) requires urgent cardioversion
    (E) is associated with a markedly increased risk of death

37. A 26-year-old patient with polycystic ovary syndrome requests treatment for her facial hirsutism. Which of the following antihypertensive medications could be prescribed?

    (A) amlodipine
    (B) propranolol
    (C) ramipril
    (D) spironolactone
    (E) clonidine

38. A 49-year-old man with a 60-pack-year history of smoking has just been diagnosed with bladder cancer. Which of the following tumors is most likely to be found on the biopsy specimens?

   (A) basal cell carcinoma
   (B) small cell carcinoma
   (C) renal cell carcinoma
   (D) pheochromocytoma
   (E) transitional cell carcinoma

39. A 42-year-old alcoholic has PCT. Which wavelength of sunlight should be avoided to avoid cutaneous outbreaks resulting from the phototoxicity?

   (A) infrared
   (B) ultraviolet A
   (C) ultraviolet B
   (D) ultraviolet C
   (E) visible

40. Pelvic fractures are

   (A) commonly seen in osteopenic elderly females
   (B) rarely associated with significant blood loss even if displaced
   (C) uncommonly associated with other injuries
   (D) infrequently seen in young athletes with muscle avulsions
   (E) most frequently seen in children

41. A graft-versus-host reaction may occur due to

   (A) a graft contaminated with gram-negative microorganisms
   (B) grafted tumor tissues
   (C) histocompability antigens not found in the recipient
   (D) immunocompetent lymphoid cells present in the graft and the recipient is immunosuppressed
   (E) tissue hypoxia

42. A 62-year-old man presents with dystrophic toenails, and a fungal culture confirms the diagnosis of onychomycosis. He is taking multiple medications putting him at risk for a drug interaction. Which of the following drugs is an inducer of cytochrome P-450?

   (A) diltiazem
   (B) erythromycin
   (C) cimetidine
   (D) itraconazole
   (E) phenytoin

43. A 34-year-old obese woman comes to the ED because of palpitations. She has had palpitations on and off for the past several months, but previously they had always subsided on their own. Her past medical history is unremarkable. She takes care of a grandmother who has hypothyroidism, and her family medical history is otherwise unremarkable. On examination, she has an irregularly irregular rhythm and is mildly diaphoretic, but without a goiter. Her blood studies reveal a suppressed thyroid-stimulating hormone (TSH). A 24-hour thyroid radioiodine uptake is performed, revealing a low uptake. A thyroglobulin level is also drawn, and this is found to be low. What is the likely cause of this patient's hyperthyroidism?

   (A) struma ovarii
   (B) exogenous (factitious) hyperthyroidism
   (C) thyroiditis
   (D) multinodular goiter
   (E) Graves' disease

44. Which of the following studies would be useful to diagnose a gastric emptying disorder?

   (A) electrogastrogram
   (B) barium swallow
   (C) abdominal radiographs
   (D) CT of the abdomen
   (E) abdominal ultrasonography

45. An elevated serum gastrin level would be unexpected in which of the following conditions?

(A) chronic renal failure

(B) Zollinger-Ellison syndrome

(C) retained gastric antrum

(D) use of proton pump inhibitors (PPIs)

(E) peptic ulcer disease

46. Which of the following is true about gastric carcinoma?

(A) Gastric cancer responds well to radiotherapy.

(B) Most patients with gastric cancer have regional lymph node metastases.

(C) The incidence of gastric cancer is decreased in patients with pernicious anemia.

(D) The incidence of gastric cancer is decreased in individuals with blood type A.

(E) The incidence of gastric cancer has been increasing in recent years.

47. Which of the following is a direct effect of insulin?

(A) stimulation of glycogen synthase

(B) increase in gluconeogenesis

(C) decrease in amino acid transport into muscles

(D) inhibition of lipoprotein lipase

(E) increase in ketogenesis

48. The most common cause of secondary amenorrhea in an 18-year-old is

(A) pituitary adenoma

(B) anorexia

(C) excessive exercise

(D) pregnancy

(E) thyroid disorder

49. A 67-year-old obese man has had poorly controlled type 2 diabetes for 15 years. He presents with the following conditions. Which of these conditions is resulting from something other than his diabetes?

(A) esophageal varices

(B) cataracts

(C) erectile dysfunction

(D) proteinuria

(E) gastroparesis

50. Stress is related to or associated with

(A) an increase in parasympathetic tone

(B) an increase in sympathetic tone

(C) hypotension

(D) paradoxical relaxation

(E) bradycardia

Answers and Explanations

1. **(A)** While barrier methods have the advantage of affording some protection against sexually transmitted diseases (STDs), they are less effective forms of birth control. Even with "perfect" use of condoms or diaphragm, a 3% to 5% 1-year failure rate is expected. This rate is even higher (15% to 20%) when typical use is studied. Copper-containing IUDs in current use are reported to have a 0.8% failure rate in 1 year of use. Combined OCs have a 0.1% failure rate.

2. **(B)** Autoimmune adrenal insufficiency is characterized by destruction of the entire adrenal cortex. Therefore, cortisol, aldosterone, and adrenal androgen levels will all be diminished, leading to a loss of the negative feedback of cortisol on the production of ACTH. Excessively elevated ACTH levels act as analogues of melanocyte-stimulating hormone and lead to hyperpigmentation. The diagnosis of primary adrenal insufficiency is confirmed by a diminished response of cortisol to ACTH stimulation (corticotropin stimulation test).

3. **(B)** There is a strong association between infection with *H. pylori* and peptic ulcer disease. Although the development of duodenal ulcers is more prevalent, the development of gastric ulcers is also possible. There is a negative association between infection with *H. pylori* and reflux esophagitis. Eradication of *H. pylori*, therefore, may result in the development of reflux esophagitis. There is no association between *H. pylori* infection and celiac disease or colorectal cancer.

4. **(D)** *Schistosoma haematobium* has been implicated in the development of bladder cancer, most often squamous cell carcinoma. In Egypt, where schistosomiasis is common among males, squamous cell cancer of the bladder is the most common malignancy.

5. **(E)** A stress test in the setting of a potential dissection could lead to a clinical catastrophe. The ECG may help detect disruption of the coronary arteries in a proximal dissection. The echocardiogram may show a proximal dissection or abnormality in the ascending aorta. It may also reveal disruption and regurgitation of the aortic valve. MRI is a noninvasive imaging procedure that uses magnetic fields and a computer to produce high-resolution cross-sectional or three-dimensional images. This is a reliable way of detecting dissections. CT is a radiographic imaging technique whereby x-ray pictures of tissues from various angles are obtained and a computer is used to consolidate the pictures to create a detailed three-dimensional cross-sectional image. Cardiac catheterization may be done to evaluate the aorta and to determine whether the coronary arteries have been disrupted. The chest x-ray may show widening of the mediastinum, suggesting aortic aneurysm or dissection.

6. **(A)** The organisms identified in the mucous layer of the gastric gland are characteristic of *H. pylori*. It is important to identify that the tissue being evaluated represents an oxyntic gland present in the stomach. It would be unusual to expect any of the other described organisms normally present in infected patients in the intestinal or colonic epithelium.

7. **(B)** In SIADH, there is hyponatremia, low plasma osmolality, and high urine osmolality.

8. **(C)** While most patients who experience infection with HPV do not develop cervical cancer, there is a strong association between cervical cancer and HPV infection. Chronic carrier status of HBV is associated with the development of liver cancer, not cervical cancer. While infection with HIV is associated with more rapid progression of precancerous cervical lesions, HPV is still believed to be a cofactor in these cases. In the past, HSV-2 was thought to be associated with cervical cancer; this is no longer believed to be true.

9. **(C)** CEA can be elevated in various tumors. However, it is most often found in patients with adenocarcinomas of the gastrointestinal tract and the pancreas.

10. **(A)** Tinea capitis is a superficial fungal infection of the scalp caused by dermatophytes. The disease varies clinically from noninflamed scaly patches to pustule-studded indurated plaques that can result in permanent scarring and hair loss.

11. **(B)** The patient has had recurrent episodes of angioedema with probable involvement of her bowels and her upper airways. The clinician should confirm that she is not on an angiotensin-converting enzyme (ACE) inhibitor, but should otherwise strongly suspect hereditary angioneurotic edema. There are two types. In type 1, there is an absolute deficiency of C1-inhibitor, while in type 2, the C1-inhibitor levels are normal or super-normal but nonfunctional. This protease is important in keeping complement activation in check by degrading the first component of the complements, but its deficiency or effective deficiency can also lead to increases in bradykinin and C2b, which leads to edema. Bone marrow biopsy may potentially identify a process like systemic mastocytosis, but the symptoms related to this are more pruritic and hallmarked by the characteristic urticaria pigmentosa. Empiric antihistamine therapy or food allergy testing would be inappropriate at this time.

12. **(C)** A type III immune complex reaction is produced by aggregations of antigen, antibody, and complement. An example of a type III reaction is cutaneous vasculitis.

13. **(D)** The sodium level should be raised slowly to avoid central pontine myelinolysis.

14. **(D)** In the overwhelming majority of cases of sexual abuse of children, the child knows the assailant. This aspect of sexual abuse of children further complicates reporting of the abuse by the child.

15. **(C)** Vitamin D stimulates absorption of calcium and phosphate from the small intestine. A deficiency of vitamin D will therefore lead to decreased absorption of both calcium and phosphate. Low levels of calcium stimulate increased levels of parathyroid hormone (PTH). The most abundant form of vitamin D, 1,25-dihydroxyvitamin D, will be diminished.

16. **(E)** Malignant melanoma most often arises in the skin but may originate in other mucosal surfaces. These tumors arise either de novo from preexisting dysplastic nevi or in familial groups. Lentigo maligna melanoma tends to arise in sun-exposed areas of the skin. Clinically, these tumors are raised lesions with irregular notched borders and may be red, white, or black or have black and brown foci. Tumors in the papillary dermis occur only as a result of direct tumor spread or recurrence. Malignant melanomas frequently metastasize either by lymphatic vessels to regional lymph nodes or hematogenously to the skin, lungs, and liver.

17. **(C)** Curettage and bone grafting also can result in healing. Unicameral cysts generally resolve by adulthood. They are the most common cause of pathologic fracture in children.

18. **(E)** Given this patient scenario, the patient likely has emphysematous pyelonephritis. This is characterized as an acute necrotizing parenchymal and perirenal infection caused by gas-forming pathogens. Women are affected more often than men. The most com-

mon organism is *E. coli*, although *Klebsiella* and *Proteus* are often seen. Xanthogranulomatous pyelonephritis is chronic renal infection, often in conjunction with obstructive uropathy secondary to lithiasis.

19. **(C)** An ultrasound would be appropriate for a palpable soft tissue mass. In the absence of positive findings in the listed tests, a CT-directed needle biopsy of the lesion would be appropriate. The most common tumor of bone is metastatic from another source.

20. **(E)** Of all the answers, treatment with a penicillin or cephalosporin is indicated. They are thought to be safe and effective in any phase of pregnancy. Tetracyclines are contraindicated because they may cause acute maternal liver decompensation and fetal malformations. Sulfa preparations may cause kernicterus and neonatal hyperbilirubinemia. The incidence of acute clinical pyelonephritis in pregnant women with bacteriuria is increased significantly, and the recommendations are to treat bacteriuria in the symptomatic or asymptomatic female in order to avoid pyelonephritis and its potential sequelae to the mother or fetus.

21. **(B)** A fracture in which bone penetrates the skin is called an open or compound fracture. A fracture comminuting with a joint is an intra-articular fracture. Twisting injuries generally produce spiral fracture patterns. A ligament or tendon bony insertion that has been pulled off is called an avulsion fracture.

22. **(C)** Glucagon stimulates glycogenolysis, gluconeogenesis, and ketogenesis, all of which antagonize the effects of insulin. Somatostatin inhibits the secretion of a variety of hormones, including insulin. Gastrin is secreted by the gastric antrum in response to ingested food and results in amplification of glucose-induced insulin release. Epinephrine and norepinephrine inhibit insulin secretion through alpha-adrenergic effects.

23. **(B)** hCG is a normal product of trophoblasts. In neoplastic disorders of trophoblasts, such as hydatidiform mole, hCG is elevated, usually beyond the levels found in normal pregnancy.

24. **(E)** OCs are effective contraceptives, with a failure rate of 2% to 3%. However, their use, as well as potential contraindications, should be carefully reviewed with the patient. These include thromboembolic diseases including stroke. Smoking, along the same lines, may potentiate a hypercoagulable state. OC use should also be avoided in women with estrogen-dependent tumors or in those at high risk for such tumors. Pregnancy is considered an absolute contraindication, although OC use early in pregnancy probably does not increase the incidence of congenital abnormalities. OCs will also worsen hypertriglyceridemia and should be avoided in such patients. Diabetes may require an increase in insulin requirements but is not a contraindication to OC use.

25. **(D)** PCT is characterized clinically by photosensitivity resulting in blister formation or erosions on sun-exposed skin. The porphyrins are a result of acquired or inherited defects in heme synthesis. Estrogens are an exogenous trigger of the disease and should be avoided.

26. **(C)** Leg ulcers and splenic infarction are common in sickle cell disease due to small vessel occlusion by sickled cells. Cholelithiasis results from hemolysis and thus increased bilirubin. Sickle cell patients are also prone to infection, and osteomyelitis is not uncommon. Pancreatitis is usually not caused by sickle cell disease but by alcohol.

27. **(E)** An association between this rare liver tumor and exposure to vinyl chloride has been established. This is a fatal tumor with little role for radiation or chemotherapy even for palliation.

28. **(C)** Fibroadenoma is the most common benign breast tumor. It is composed of connective tissue with ductal and acinar elements. The other options occur much less frequently.

29. (B) The clinical picture most likely represents polycystic ovary syndrome (PCOS). It is generally a diagnosis of exclusion, and the differential includes other causes of hyperandrogenism. An abrupt onset later in life is typical for some of these rare disorders that include prolactinomas, ovarian tumors, congenital adrenal hyperplasia, and adrenal tumors. PCOS presents around the peripubertal time with oligomenorrhea or amenorrhea. Androgen and testosterone levels are frequently elevated. As many as 35% of these patients will have glucose intolerance of varying severity (including diabetes). Although most patients with PCOS do have eight or more follicles per each ovary (polycystic ovaries), the diagnosis is not dependent on the radiographic presence of these cystic ovaries.

30. (B) In the majority of cirrhotic patients with spontaneous bacterial peritonitis, the most common enteric organism is *E. coli*. Among nonenteric organisms, *Listeria monocytogenes* is the most common. The most common anaerobic organism identified in cultures is *Bacteroides* species.

31. (B) DHEA-S comes mainly from the adrenals. When it is very high, imaging of the adrenals should be performed in order to exclude an adrenal neoplasm.

32. (D) VLDL contains the highest concentration of triglycerides, followed by IDL, LDL, HDL, and Lp(a), which contain cholesteryl esters as their primary core lipids.

33. (D) Thrombin has a specificity for arginine–glycine bonds similar to trypsin. Thrombin is synthesized as prothrombin, which contains gamma-carboxyglutamate residues deriving from vitamin K–dependent post-translational modification of glutamate. In order to be activated, prothromin is proteolytically cleaved by factor Xa after being anchored to platelet membranes in a calcium gamma-carboxyglutamate–dependent reaction.

34. (A) Type I anaphylactic reactions are caused by the combination of allergens with immunoglobulin E (IgE) molecules on mast cells and basophils. An example of a type I reaction is urticaria.

35. (A) A pure anmestic syndrome is more typical of Korsakoff's syndrome. Thiamine replacement may produce improvement in the symptoms of Wernicke's syndrome, but the amnestic syndrome of Korsakoff's syndrome is typically resistant to therapy. Wernicke's syndrome (from thiamine deficiency) may present with choices B, C, D, and E.

36. (B) Atrial fibrillation occurs when the sinus node is no longer functioning as the primary pacemaker of the heart. It is associated with a variety of cardiac conditions but can occur in a structurally normal heart. The AV node serves to prevent the rapid atrial activity from reaching the ventricles and thereby plays a protective role. There is increased mortality associated over time with atrial fibrillation, but that increase is slight. The prognosis of atrial fibrillation is largely related to the underlying cardiac condition. Stroke or embolism is the major negative consequence of atrial fibrillation, and patients at risk for stroke should be anticoagulated.

37. (D) Spironolactone has antiandrogenic properties.

38. (E) Transitional cell carcinoma has a fourfold higher incidence in smokers compared to nonsmokers. The exact causative agent is yet to be found, although 4-aminobiphenyl has been implicated. Squamous cell carcinoma of the bladder is usually seen in *Schistosoma* infections and chronic catheterization. Small cell carcinoma and pheomchromocytomas are exceedingly rare and not definitively linked to cigarette smoking. Renal cell carcinoma is not found in the bladder.

39. (E) The porphyrins show peak absorption in the 400–410-nm region, also known as the Soret band, which is in the visible spectrum. It is postulated that the sunlight creates excited-state porphyrin molecules that transfer energy to oxygen molecules, and these reactive oxygen species inflict tissue damage. Because the putative wavelengths are in the visible spectrum, physical sunblocks are necessary for photoprotection.

40. **(A)** Most pelvic fractures are nondisplaced fractures seen in elderly females with osteopenic bone. Pelvic fractures in younger patients and even children are usually the result of high-energy trauma and are associated with significant blood loss and other severe injuries. Avulsion fractures involving the insertion of the sartorius muscle on the anterior superior iliac spine are common in younger athletes.

41. **(D)** The graft-versus-host reaction occurs when immunocompetent lymphoid cells (T cells) are transferred to a histoincompatible recipient who is unable to reject them. The donor cells then mount an immune response against the foreign histocompatibility antigens of the recipient and attempt to reject them.

42. **(E)** Cytochrome P-450 is a family of enzymes predominantly abundant in the liver that oxidize a large number of drugs. Drug interactions frequently occur when drugs are administered simultaneously, and one drug affects the metabolic clearance of the other by inducing or inhibiting enzymatic activity. Phenytoin is an important inducer of cytochrome P-450, while the other drugs listed are inhibitors.

43. **(B)** The patient has hyperthyroidism based on her clinical presentation and the suppressed TSH. The reduced thyroid radioiodine uptake narrows the differential considerably to either exogenous hyperthyroidism, ectopic hyperthyroid tissue, a subacute thyroiditis, or an iodine-induced hyperthyroidism. If the radioiodine uptake were to be taken over the area of a potential ectopic hyperthyroid tissue (such as a struma ovarii), the uptake would be increased. The serum thyroglobulin level further reduces the differ-

ential to exogenous hyperthyroidism alone, as the other causes listed would be reflected by increased levels. The patient has access to levothyroxine from her grandmother and may very well have been surreptitiously taking this for weight loss, for example.

44. **(A)** Of the tests listed, only an electrogastrogram would provide useful information regarding the etiology of a gastric motility disorder. A barium swallow would study only the esophagus. CT or ultrasonography, although useful studies to evaluate for anatomic abnormalities, would not provide functional information.

45. **(E)** Of the conditions listed, only peptic ulcer disease is not generally associated with an elevation in the serum gastrin level. Serum gastrin becomes elevated in chronic renal failure because the kidneys are the primary site of excretion of the gastrin hormone. Zollinger-Ellison syndrome is associated with elevations in the serum gastrin level owing to the release of the hormone by a gastrinoma tumor. Similarly, the retained antrum syndrome occurs in patients who undergo a gastric resection and a remnant of antral tissue remains, containing the G cells and thus releasing gastrin, which cannot be inhibited by the release of acid. The use of PPIs is well associated with the development of modest elevations in serum gastrin due to the lack of negative feedback inhibition by acid secretion.

46. **(B)** The incidence of gastric cancer has been declining in the Western world. Those with blood group A and achlorhydria from atrophic gastritis or pernicious anemia are at increased risk for gastric cancer. The tumor often presents with locoregional spread. In general, gastric cancer is not a good radioresponder, and trials using concurrent chemotherapy with radiation are under way to control the disease both locally and distantly.

47. **(A)** The major function of insulin is to promote storage of nutrients. Insulin promotes

the storage of glucose as glycogen by stimulating glycogen synthase, inhibits the conversion of amino acids to glucose (inhibits gluconeogenesis), increases the transport of amino acids into muscle, and inhibits the conversion of fatty acids and amino acids to ketoacids. It also stimulates lipoprotein lipase, which causes the hydrolysis of triglycerides from circulating lipoproteins.

48. **(D)** While anorexia, excessive exercise, and a prolactin-secreting pituitary adenoma can all cause secondary amenorrhea, by far the most common cause is pregnancy in women in the reproductive age group.

49. **(A)** Esophageal varices are a result of portal hypertension, which is usually due to hepatic cirrhosis and is not a complication of diabetes. Cataracts are a complication of diabetes and may be due to glycosylation of lens protein and an excess of lenticular sorbitol. Erectile dysfunction in diabetes is due to neuropathy and peripheral vascular disease. Gastroparesis is seen in diabetes and is a result of autonomic neuropathy. The diabetic kidney develops glomerulosclerosis and proteinuria, eventually leading to renal failure.

50. **(B)** Stress is a physical and emotional response. The change could be anything from financial pressures to heavy traffic. Different people feel stress from different situations. Significant emotional stress can generate an increase in the sympathetic tone or a "fight-or-flight" response. This affects the immune system and the digestive system as well as the cardiovascular system. The heart rate and blood pressure increase, and the metabolic rate is accelerated. Frequent or lasting periods of significant emotional stress have been associated with an increased risk of hypertension, arrhythmias, and elevated cholesterol levels. Stress has been linked to an increased risk of heart attack and stroke.

Practice Test 13
Questions

DIRECTIONS (Questions 1 through 50): Each of the numbered items or incomplete statements in this section is followed by answers or by completions of the statement. Select the ONE lettered answer or completion that is BEST in each case.

1. A patient who has a known 46,XY karyotype and complete androgen resistance presents to you for evaluation. Which of the following statements is true regarding this syndrome?

   (A) The patient will have ovaries in place of testes.
   (B) The patient will have external female genitalia.
   (C) The patient will have diminished testosterone levels.
   (D) The patient will have a uterus.
   (E) The patient will lack estradiol.

2. Vertigo that worsens with head turning is most suggestive of an abnormality of the

   (A) cochlea
   (B) vestibular nerve
   (C) pons
   (D) cerebellum
   (E) auditory cortex

3. Which of the following is a peptide hormone that binds to a seven-transmembrane domain receptor?

   (A) thyroid-stimulating hormone (TSH)
   (B) triiodothyronine (T_3)
   (C) 1,25-dihydroxyvitamin D
   (D) estradiol
   (E) luteinizing hormone (LH) receptor

4. Allergic contact dermatitis is an example of which type of immune reaction?

   (A) type I
   (B) type II
   (C) type III
   (D) type IV
   (E) type V

5. The ophthalmoscopic finding in Figure 13.1 may be seen in

   (A) frontal lobe meningioma
   (B) occipital lobe stroke
   (C) acute optic neuritis
   (D) diabetic retinopathy
   (E) temporal arteritis

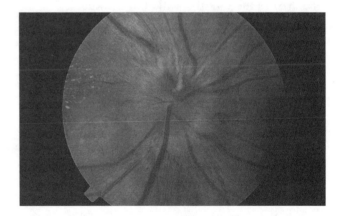

Figure 13.1

6. Following a fracture of the middle third of the humerus, the radial nerve is observed not to be functioning. Which of the following is true?

(A) Wrist extension is present but not metacarpophalangeal (MCP) extension.

(B) Both wrist and MCP extension are present.

(C) Wrist and MCP extension are present, and the patient cannot extend the interphalangeal (IP) joints.

(D) There may be decreased sensation in the anatomic snuffbox area.

(E) Strength and motion will not be affected.

7. Beneficial effects of alcohol may include

(A) decreasing uptake of low-density lipoprotein (LDL)

(B) increasing high-density lipoprotein (HDL)

(C) oxidating of LDL

(D) antiplatelet activity

(E) preventing coronary constriction

8. The best description of the x-ray in Figure 13.2 is

(A) an anterior dislocation of the knee

(B) a medial dislocation of the knee

(C) a lateral dislocation of the knee

(D) a posterior dislocation of the knee

(E) a dislocation of the patella

9. Which of the following statements is true regarding the effects of diabetes?

(A) Blood vessel damage related to hyperglycemia contributes to the thickening of the walls.

(B) Plaque growth is unaffected in diabetes.

(C) Coronary artery disease (CAD) progression is retarded by the antioxidant effects of lowered LDL in diabetes.

(D) Cardiomyopathy does not occur because of restricted blood flow due to inflammation of the heart muscle.

(E) Very few diabetic patients die from heart or blood vessel disease.

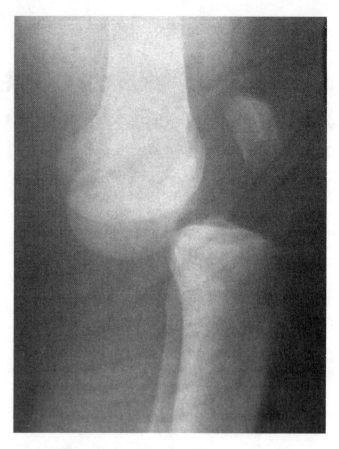

Figure 13.2
(Reprinted, with permission, from *Campbell's Operative Orthopaedics*, 9th ed., p. 2634.)

10. A 42-year-old man presents to your clinic desiring a referral for a circumcision. He inquires about the subsequent risk of developing penile cancer. You tell him that

(A) circumcision increases the risk of penile cancer

(B) circumcision decreases the risk of penile cancer

(C) there is no difference in the risk of penile cancer

(D) it is unknown if there is any change in risk

(E) risk is linked to the amount of tissue removed

11. A lacunar stroke is most likely to be due to occlusion of the

    (A) anterior cerebral artery
    (B) middle cerebral artery
    (C) posterior cerebral artery
    (D) lenticulostriate artery
    (E) vertebral artery

12. Annually, what percentage of pregnancies in the United States are unintended?

    (A) 20%
    (B) 80%
    (C) 50%
    (D) 10%
    (E) 90%

13. You examine a 28-year-old woman who is found to have a lesion in the hypothalamus. Which endocrine disorder is resulting from a condition other than the hypothalamic lesion?

    (A) diabetes mellitus
    (B) adrenal insufficiency
    (C) hyperprolactinemia
    (D) diabetes insipidus
    (E) hypothyroidism

14. Head and neck cancers are associated with

    (A) dye and printing chemicals
    (B) asbestos
    (C) ulcerative colitis
    (D) Epstein-Barr virus
    (E) pernicious anemia

15. What is the most likely diagnosis of the patient shown in Figure 13.3?

    (A) psoriasis
    (B) varicella
    (C) folliculitis
    (D) vitiligo
    (E) Kaposi's sarcoma

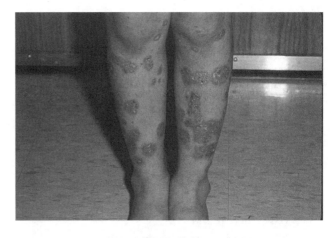

Figure 13.3

16. Which of the following statements is true regarding ruptured cerebral artery aneurysms?

    (A) Spinal fluid analysis is always abnormal.
    (B) Computed tomography (CT) scan of the head is always abnormal.
    (C) Oculomotor nerve palsy is not a presenting sign.
    (D) They do not arise from bifurcations within the circle of Willis.
    (E) They are not associated with hereditary renal disease.

17. In diabetics

    (A) the incidence of stroke is no greater than in the general population
    (B) atherosclerosis is 50 times more common than in nondiabetics
    (C) circulation is affected only in large blood vessels
    (D) major organs of the body may not get enough oxygen-rich blood because of direct effects of hyperglycemia
    (E) moderate insulin deficiency indicates a higher risk of heart disease

18. A 12-year-old boy presents following a 10-foot fall from a tree. He has an obvious fracture of the right tibia. The leg has good distal pulses and normal sensory and motor function. The skin over the fracture is intact. His blood pressure is 110/70, and his pulse is 90. He is complaining of severe leg pain, which has been unresponsive to splinting of his fracture and parenteral morphine sulfate. The most likely cause of his pain is

(A) compartment syndrome
(B) fracture pain
(C) unrecognized lumbar spine injury with nerve root compression
(D) intimal tear of the posterior tibial artery with resulting ischemic leg pain
(E) phantom limb pain

19. Which of the following infectious agents is known to result in a respiratory illness?

(A) human papillomavirus (HPV)
(B) *Treponema pallidum*
(C) hepatitis B virus (HBV)
(D) *Chlamydia psittaci*
(E) *Haemophilus ducreyi*

20. A 26-year-old woman presents with tachycardia, weight loss, and tremors. She is found to be hyperthyroid. She undergoes a radioactive iodine uptake and scan. During this test, she is given a pill containing radioactive iodine. The degree of iodine trapping by the thyroid gland is then assessed quantitatively. In which of the following conditions would the thyroid gland exhibit decreased uptake of iodine?

(A) Graves' disease
(B) toxic thyroid nodule
(C) TSH-secreting adenoma
(D) exogenous thyroid hormone intake
(E) euthyroid patient

21. Bladder carcinoma is linked to

(A) dye and printing chemicals
(B) asbestos
(C) ulcerative colitis

(D) EBV
(E) pernicious anemia

22. Which of the following hormone–target cell pairs is correct?

(A) luteinizing hormone (LH)–Sertoli cell
(B) follicle-stimulating hormone (FSH)–Leydig cell
(C) FSH–theca cell
(D) human chorionic gonadotropin (hCG)–luteal cell
(E) FSH–luteal cell

23. Anemia is one of several complications following Billroth II gastrectomy for peptic ulcer disease. Which of the following may contribute to anemia?

(A) dumping syndrome
(B) iron malabsorption and vitamin B_{12} malabsorption
(C) avoiding multivitamin use
(D) lack of red meat in the diet
(E) excess fiber in the diet

24. A 30-year-old man develops diffuse flushing and severe dyspnea following a bee sting. On arrival at the emergency department (ED), he is found to be hypotensive and has diffuse wheezing on auscultation of his chest. Urticaria can be seen scattered on his trunk. Which of the following immune-related mechanisms plays an integral role in the initiation of this hypersensitivity reaction?

(A) immune complex formation
(B) deficiency or dysfunction of C1-esterase inhibitor
(C) immunoglobulin E (IgE) cross-linkage on mast cells
(D) anaphylactoid reaction
(E) T cell–mediated cytotoxicity

25. In response to a viral infection in a healthy adolescent, which of the following cell types, when infected with the virus, is able to present peptide fragments of the virus for recognition by antigen-specific CD8+ cytotoxic T cells?

(A) platelets

(B) gametes

(C) erythrocytes

(D) neurons

(E) eosinophils

26. Budd-Chiari syndrome is caused by obstruction of the

(A) superior vena cava

(B) portal vein

(C) hepatic vein

(D) splenic vein

(E) aorta

27. A 40-year-old nonsmoker has developed severe emphysema due to alpha$_1$-antitrypsin deficiency. Which of the following phenotypes of the alpha$_1$-antitrypsin is likely in this patient and would not predispose this man to the development of cirrhosis of the liver?

(A) PI*MM

(B) PI*null-null

(C) PI*ZZ

(D) PI*OB

(E) PI*OA

28. The photomicrograph obtained from a gastric mucosal biopsy in the body of the stomach as shown in Figure 13.4 demonstrates

(A) parietal cell hyperplasia

(B) chief cell hyperplasia

(C) carcinoid tumor

(D) gastric carcinoma

(E) glandular tumor

29. Lyme disease is caused by

(A) *Borrelia burgdorferi*

(B) *Rickettsia akari*

(C) *Rickettsia quintana*

(D) *Ancylostoma brasiliense*

(E) *Ehrlichia canis*

30. Which of the following is the primary effector cell of an immediate hypersensitivity reaction?

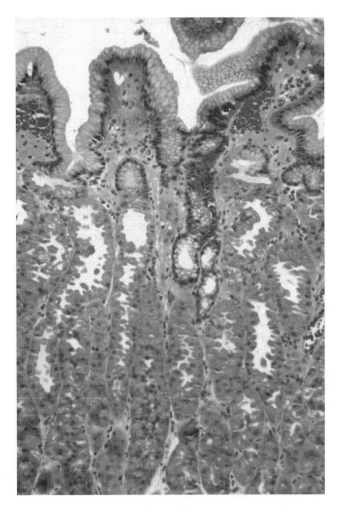

Figure 13.4

(A) eosinophil

(B) mast cell

(C) red blood cell (RBC)

(D) neutrophil

(E) T lymphocyte

31. A 45-year-old woman presents to the ED with a gradual onset of increasing headaches and right-sided weakness. A CT scan is obtained, with no evidence of a vascular event but with a lesion noted. Which of the following may be responsible?

(A) malignant lymphoma

(B) ependymoma

(C) glioblastoma multiforme

(D) meningioma

(E) mesothelioma

32. What is the mode of *Babesia* transmission?

    (A) dog tick (*Dermacentor variabilis*) or wood tick (*Dermacentor andersoni*)
    (B) deer tick (*Ixodes scapularis*)
    (C) *Borrelia burgdorferi*
    (D) *Treponema pallidum*
    (E) *Rickettsia rickettsii*

33. A 55-year-old man presents with a 3-month history of severe headache, double vision, and seizures. Which of the following central nervous system (CNS) lesions may be responsible?

    (A) meningioma
    (B) malignant lymphoma
    (C) ependymoma
    (D) progressive multifocal leukodystrophy
    (E) glioblastoma multiforme

34. At what age does fetal urine contribute to amniotic fluid?

    (A) 10 weeks
    (B) 15 weeks
    (C) 21 weeks
    (D) 27 weeks
    (E) weeks 2–3

35. Meralgia paresthetica is associated with the

    (A) median nerve within the carpal tunnel
    (B) ulnar nerve within the cubital tunnel
    (C) oculomotor nerve
    (D) lateral femoral cutaneous nerve
    (E) phrenic nerve

36. A 55-year-old man is admitted after a drug overdose and is intubated. He is initially placed on assist-control mode on the ventilator with a respiratory rate of 12, tidal volume of 500 mL, fraction of inspired oxygen (FiO_2) of 100% and a positive end-expiratory pressure (PEEP) of 5. His blood gas is as follows: pH 7.24, PCO_2 60, PO_2 300. Which of the following are the two modalities that, when changed, will significantly affect the acid–base status?

    (A) FiO_2 and PEEP
    (B) tidal volume and FiO_2
    (C) PEEP and respiratory rate
    (D) tidal volume and respiratory rate
    (E) PEEP and FiO_2

37. The urinary bladder is derived primarily from

    (A) endoderm
    (B) mesoderm
    (C) endoderm and mesoderm
    (D) endoderm and ectoderm
    (E) ectoderm

38. Which of the following structures is contained in the femoral triangle?

    (A) vastus lateralis
    (B) sartorius
    (C) inguinal ligament
    (D) adductor longus
    (E) femoral nerve, artery, and vein

39. An 80-year-old woman presents with sudden pain in her left lower extremity. Examination reveals an irregularly irregular rhythm. Her left leg is cool, pale, and pulseless as compared to the other leg. What will provide this patient with definitive therapy for her acute symptoms?

    (A) intravenous heparin therapy
    (B) vasodilators
    (C) embolectomy
    (D) fasciotomy
    (E) venous ultrasound

40. Which of the following is true regarding Depo-Provera?

    (A) predictable bleeding
    (B) no delay in resumption of fertility after discontinuation of medication
    (C) lack of protection against sexually transmitted diseases (STDs)
    (D) less than 85% effectiveness
    (E) no side effects

41. A 48-year-old previously healthy man is admitted to the hospital with acute left lower extremity edema and pain following a prolonged flight. He has no prior medical history and denies both prior hospitalizations and surgeries. An ultrasound confirms an acute deep venous thrombosis (DVT), and intravenous heparin is initiated. On hospital day 6, an acute severe thrombocytopenia develops. What is the next most appropriate step?

    (A) platelet transfusion
    (B) intravenous steroids
    (C) discontinue heparin and consider alternatives
    (D) inferior vena caval filter placement
    (E) fresh frozen plasma

42. Hormone replacement therapy (HRT) after menopause is indicated for the treatment of

    (A) vasomotor symptoms
    (B) hair loss
    (C) weight gain
    (D) prevention of endometrial cancer
    (E) vaginal bleeding

Questions 43 through 45

A 35-year-old man is prepared for a bronchoscopy with small doses of a short-acting benzodiazepine and some topical anesthetics (benzocaine). The procedure is uncomplicated, but shortly after completion of the bronchoscopy, the patient develops central cyanosis and a pulse oximeter saturation of 84%. An arterial blood gas (ABG) immediately drawn while on room air reveals a pH of 7.44, $PaCO_2$ 34, PaO_2 98, and a measured saturation of 81%.

43. What test should be done to reveal the diagnosis?

    (A) repeat ABG on 100% oxygen
    (B) repeat ABG from a different site to ensure it was not a venous sample
    (C) check the pulse oximetry sitting and standing
    (D) chest x-ray and a ventilation–perfusion (V/Q) scan
    (E) multiple wavelength co-oximetery

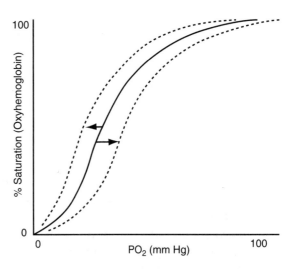

Figure 13.5

44. What is the indicated treatment for this patient?

    (A) noninvasive positive pressure ventilation and consideration of endotracheal intubation
    (B) methylene blue 1 to 2 mg/kg IV
    (C) heparin bolus at 80 units/kg IV
    (D) hyperbaric oxygen
    (E) flumazenil

45. In this patient, which direction will the oxygen–hemoglobin dissociation curve shift (see Figure 13.5)?

    (A) right
    (B) left
    (C) no change
    (D) unable to determine
    (E) the curve will flatten

46. Which is the primary collagen found in cartilage?

    (A) type I
    (B) type II
    (C) type III
    (D) type IV
    (E) type V

47. Which of the following is a cutaneous manifestation of tuberous sclerosis?

    (A) acrochordon
    (B) subungual fibroma
    (C) alopecia
    (D) acanthosis nigricans
    (E) aphthous ulcer

48. A 6-month-old female infant presents to the ED with seizures. There was no preceding illness of any sort, and she is noted to have scattered areas of decreased pigmentation on the upper back. What is the most likely diagnosis?

    (A) neurofibromatosis
    (B) incontinentia pigmenti
    (C) tuberous sclerosis
    (D) vitiligo
    (E) tinea versicolor

49. Multiple endocrine neoplasia type 1 (MEN 1) is associated with most of the following clinical syndromes. Which syndrome is associated with MEN 2?

    (A) pituitary adenomas
    (B) increase in serum calcium
    (C) hyperparathyroidism
    (D) pheochromocytomas
    (E) pancreatic islet cell tumors

50. The Blalock-Taussig procedure involves

    (A) closure of a ventricular septal defect (VSD)
    (B) creation of an atrial septal defect (ASD) by septostomy
    (C) creating a shunt from the right atrium to the pulmonary artery
    (D) creating a shunt from the aorta to the pulmonary artery
    (E) being performed around the age of 8 years

Answers and Explanations

1. **(B)** Complete androgen resistance (testicular feminization) is caused by absent or defective androgen receptors. During embryogenesis, the embryonic gonads of a genotypic male differentiate as testes under the influence of the SRY and other genes. The testicular Sertoli cells secrete anti-müllerian hormone, which inhibits the differentiation of the müllerian ducts into the fallopian tubes, the cervix, and the corpus of the uterus. In the absence of testosterone or of functioning testosterone receptors, the fetus will develop female external genitalia. Testicular Leydig cells produce testosterone, and these levels will be elevated. Estradiol is produced by the testes and by the peripheral conversion of testosterone and androstenedione.

2. **(B)** Positional vertigo usually suggests a peripheral localization and may be seen in dysfunction of the labyrinth as well as the vestibular nerve. The nystagmus is typically rotatory in appearance. Common etiologies include recent viral infection, small-vessel ischemia, or trauma, but when recurrent over years, may suggest a diagnosis of benign positional vertigo.

3. **(A)** TSH is a peptide hormone that binds to a seven-transmembrane domain receptor that activates both the G protein–adenylyl cyclase–cyclic adenosine monophosphate (cAMP) and phospholipase C cascades. T_3, 1,25-dihydroxyvitamin D, and estradiol exert their effects through binding to a nuclear receptor.

4. **(D)** Allergic contact dermatitis is a type 4 delayed hypersensitivity reaction. An example is an allergic reaction to poison ivy.

5. **(A)** Papilledema is commonly seen in frontal lobe meningioma, brain abscess, pseudotumor cerebri, and cortical vein thrombosis, but must be distinguished from acute optic neuritis (as seen in multiple sclerosis). The etiology is felt to be due to increased intracranial pressure that is transmitted to the optic nerve sheaths with subsequent blockage of venous return from the retina and optic disk. Visual acuity is typically normal in early papilledema, with later development of an enlarged blind spot with increased swelling of the optic nerve head.

6. **(D)** Wrist and MCP joint extension and sensation in the anatomic snuffbox are controlled by the radial nerve. IP joint extension is the function of the lumbrical muscles innervated by the median and ulnar nerves.

7. **(A)** Alcohol may have specific heart-related benefits. These include raising the HDL and lowering blood pressure. Alcohol may have an antioxidant effect that helps reduce damage caused by LDL oxidation. Alcohol may have antiplatelet activity and may help prevent the constriction of coronary arteries.

8. **(A)** A dislocation is described by the position of the distal half of the joint. A dislocation of the knee is a true emergency due to the potential disruption of the popliteal artery.

9. **(A)** Hyperglycemia directly damages blood vessels, contributing to thickening of their walls and acceleration of buildup of fatty materials in the blood vessels. Plaque growth is accelerated. CAD and peripheral vascular disease are accelerated. Cardiomyopathy can occur as a result of restricted blood flow due to inflammation of the heart muscle. Two thirds of diabetic patients die from heart or blood vessel disease.

10. **(C)** Circumcision has been well established as a measure that virtually eliminates the occurrence of penile carcinoma when performed at an early age. However, adult circumcision appears to offer little or no additional protection.

11. **(D)** Lacunar strokes arise from occlusion of the small perforating blood vessels, which are given off the larger cerebral vessels mentioned in the other choices. These small arteries develop lipohyalinosis and Charcot-Bouchard microaneurysms in the setting of such systemic diseases as hypertension. The most common anatomic locations for these deep, subcortical infarctions are internal capsule, thalamus, cerebellum, and pons.

12. **(C)** According to several reports surveying American women, about half of the pregnancies that occur in America are unplanned. Because of this, many groups recommend that all women of reproductive age be counseled about healthy prepregnancy behaviors such as the daily consumption of 0.4 mg of folic acid and avoidance of excessive alcohol consumption.

13. **(A)** Diabetes mellitus does not result from a hypothalamic lesion. Adrenal insufficiency may occur secondary to corticotropin-releasing hormone (CRH) deficiency, leading to diminished corticotropin and cortisol levels. The hypothalamus secretes dopamine, which inhibits prolactin secretion. Therefore, diminished dopamine production may lead to hyperprolactinemia. The nerve terminals in the posterior pituitary gland originate in the hypothalamus, and a lesion in this region may result in antidiuretic hormone (ADH) deficiency or diabetes insipidus. Diminished thyrotropin-releasing hormone (TRH) may lead to hypothyroidism.

14. **(D)** In general, the leading risk factors for head/neck cancers are tobacco and alcohol. However, in the absence of those risk factors, Epstein-Barr virus has been linked to a less common form of head/neck cancer, nasopharyngeal carcinoma, but with the advent of polymerase chain reaction (PCR), EBV is now also being seen in a cohort of classic squamous cell head/neck cancers.

15. **(A)** Psoriasis is characterized by sharply demarcated, erythematous plaques with silvery scales.

16. **(A)** CT scan of the head may miss 10 to 15% of subarachnoid hemorrhages from ruptured aneurysm, and lumbar puncture should be pursued if there is a strong clinical suspicion. Xanthochromia may be seen along with grossly bloody spinal fluid that does not resolve when measured in serial specimens. The third cranial nerve may be compressed by posterior communicating artery aneurysms. Polycystic kidney disease may be associated with familial cerebral aneurysms.

17. **(E)** Heart attack and stroke are more common in diabetics than in the general population. Atherosclerosis is up to six times more common in diabetics than in nondiabetics. Diabetes can interfere with circulation in both large and small blood vessels. This results in damage to major organs of the body. Even moderate insulin deficiency indicates a higher risk of heart disease.

18. **(A)** Compartment syndrome occurs when the interstitial pressure exceeds the closing pressure of venous outflow secondary to hemorrhage and soft tissue edema. Increasing pressure closes off arterioles and capillaries. Muscle fascia does not allow dissipation of this pressure. If allowed to continue, usually more than 6 hours, muscle cell death occurs. The signs are swelling with firmness of

the involved muscle groups, pain unresponsive to narcotic medication and splinting or fracture repair, and severe pain in the involved muscle groups to passive flexion and extension of the digits. The diagnosis is confirmed with pressure measurement of the involved compartment with a catheter connected to an arterial pressure monitor. The treatment is emergent release of the fascia covering the involved muscle group or groups. The resulting wounds are later closed primarily or covered with skin grafts after swelling has subsided.

19. **(D)** *Chlamydia trachomatis* is associated with sexually transmitted cervicitis and pelvic inflammatory disease as well as lymphogranuloma venereum. *Treponema pallidum* is the organism that causes syphilis. The sexually transmitted HPV causes genital warts. The most common mode of transmission of HBV is sexual. *Haemophilus ducreyi* causes chancroid, an STD that is uncommon in the United States. *Chlamydia psittaci* is a common infectious disease of birds and can cause severe respiratory illness in humans.

20. **(D)** TSH stimulates the uptake of iodine by the thyroid cell. Therefore, TSH-secreting adenomas would lead to increased uptake of radioactive iodine by the thyroid gland. Graves' disease is associated with TSH receptor–stimulating antibodies. This disease is thus associated with an increased uptake of radioactive iodine. Toxic nodules are autonomous and trap iodine. Exogenous thyroid hormone inhibits the release of TSH from the pituitary gland, which leads to decreased uptake of radioactive iodine by the thyroid.

21. **(A)** Bladder cancers have been linked to tobacco as well as certain chemical and biologic carcinogens. There is a well-documented association between occupational exposure to dye and printing chemicals and the development of bladder tumors.

22. **(D)** LH stimulates the ovarian theca cells to synthesize androgens. FSH stimulates the ovarian granulosa cells to convert the androgens to estrogens and to synthesize other maturational proteins. LH stimulates the testicular Leydig cells to secrete testosterone, whereas FSH stimulates the testicular Sertoli cells to secrete anti-müllerian hormone, androgen-binding protein, and other maturational proteins. During pregnancy, hCG maintains the corpus luteum's ability to secrete estrogen and progesterone.

23. **(B)** Anemia can occur in 25% of patients after peptic ulcer surgery. Iron absorption is poor because of a lack of gastric acid. Vitamin B_{12} absorption is also poor. Inflammation in the remaining portion of the stomach is a common postsurgical problem and may be due to bile in the gastric pouch and may lead to chronic gastritis with chronic low-grade blood loss. Dumping syndrome can cause weakness but does not contribute to anemia.

24. **(C)** Anaphylaxis is an IgE-mediated immediate hypersensitivity reaction (type I) that occurs in response to a reexposure to a foreign antigen. IgE formed from the initial exposures recognizes the antigen on reexposure, leading to cross-linkage of IgE on mast cells. This initiates the release of primary and secondary mediators from mast cells and basophils, including histamine, tryptase, prostaglandins, leukotrienes, platelet-activating factors, and other proinflammatory cytokines. These act in concert to promote vasodilation, vascular permeability, and bronchial smooth muscle contractions, leading to the clinical syndrome of anaphylaxis. Anaphylactoid reactions are clinically identical in their initial presentation to anaphylaxis but are mediated by a nonimmune (non-IgE-mediated) mechanism.

25. **(A)** Class I major histocompatibility complex (MHC) is found in nearly all cell types except for gametes, erythrocytes, cells of the trophoblast, and neurons. They play an integral role in allowing the immune system to recognize infected cells. Foreign proteins are processed into short peptides and expressed on the cell membrane attached to the class I

MHC. This allows recognition of the infected cell by CD8+ cytotoxic T lymphocytes, which then initates the cascade, leading to the destruction of the infected cell.

26. **(C)** The general symptom complex associated with this disorder is that of ascites and hepatomegaly. Thrombosis, intimal fibrosis, or tumor involvement of the hepatic veins or inferior vena cava can result in this syndrome. The portal and splenic veins are patent in this condition.

27. **(C)** Alpha$_1$-antitrypsin inhibits the action of neutrophil elastase. Its deficiency—and therefore the unchecked activity of elastase in the lungs—favors the development of premature panacinar emphysema. However, the etiology of liver disease in patients with alpha$_1$-antitrypsin deficiency is not related to the unchecked activity of elastase. Rather, it is the accumulation of the dysfunctional alpha$_1$-antitrypsin in the endoplasmic reticulum of hepatocytes that is felt to lead to liver injury and potentially cirrhosis. Therefore, the "null" alleles, implying complete absence of any alpha$_1$-antitrypsin, should not cause liver dysfunction, as there is no abnormal alpha$_1$-antitrypsin to accumulate in the liver. However, its deficiency is absolute, and therefore lung disease can still develop. The "M" allele is normal, and its homozygous expression would not lead to liver disease, but would also not lead to alpha$_1$-antitrypsin deficiency–associated emphysema as in our patient. The phenotypic expression of the homozygous "Z" allele is the most common cause of clinically significant alpha$_1$-antitrypsin deficiency.

28. **(A)** The photomicrograph shows an increase in the numbers of parietal cells that are present, consistent with parietal cell hyperplasia taken from a patient on chronic proton pump inhibitor (PPI) therapy.

29. **(A)** Erythema migrans is the most diagnostic manifestation of Lyme disease, a tick-borne illness caused by the spirochete *Borrelia burgdorferi.*

30. **(B)** Type I anaphylactic reactions are caused by the combination of allergens with IgE molecules on mast cells and basophils.

31. **(D)** Meningiomas are slow-growing tumors, and the slow progression of neurological problems may be consistent with this tumor. They generally arise in the arachnoid covering of the brain and are considered benign. Patients with meningiomas usually present with seizures, hemiparesis, visual field loss, aphasia, or cranial nerve abnormalities. They enhance on CT with contrast. The treatment of choice is resection.

32. **(B)** *Babesia* can be carried by the *Ixodes* tick. This is the same tick that carries *Borrelia burgdorferi,* the spirochete that is the cause of Lyme disease.

33. **(E)** Glioblastoma multiforme is a fairly rapidly growing CNS lesion seen in men. The lesion described in the question indicates this lesion, but this will have to be biopsy proven. The role of surgery is to secure a diagnosis, alleviate symptoms related to intracranial pressure or compression, and recue the need for steroids. The median survival is generally 4 to 6 months. Radiation therapy does have a small survival advantage and the role of chemotherapy is marginal; thus, most patients are now enrolled in clinical trials.

34. **(A)** The permanent fetal kidneys begin to develop early in the fifth week and start to produce urine about 4 to 5 weeks later.

35. **(D)** Diabetes may commonly be associated with choices A through D. Carpal tunnel syndrome may be seen in 40% of diabetic patients. Lateral femoral cutaneous neuropathy (numbness of the lateral aspect of the thigh) may also be seen in such conditions as pregnancy or obesity. It is typically associated with a burning, hyperesthetic pain and is then called *meralgia paresthetica.*

36. **(D)** Mechanical ventilation is often used in critically ill patients. One ventilator mode, assist control, has four main components that

the practitioner can set: FiO_2, PEEP, tidal volume, and respiratory rate. The tidal volume and respiratory rate are primarily responsible for acid–base exchange. The FiO_2 and PEEP are primarily responsible for the patient's oxygenation—how much oxygen they are inhaling and the pressure at the level of the alveoli. Oxygenation is improved when the end-expiratory pressure is increased at the level of the alveoli (PEEP), thereby helping with oxygen exchange at that level. The patient has respiratory acidosis, and decreasing the CO_2 by either increasing the respiratory rate or the tidal volume will help normalize the pH. When a patient has trouble oxygenating, inhaled oxygen can be increased, but not above 100%. If improved oxygenation is needed at an FiO_2 of 100%, the PEEP can be increased. This can help oxygenation at the alveolar level. (The blood pressure should be watched carefully as it can decrease as the PEEP is increased.)

37. **(C)** The epithelium of the bladder is derived from the endoderm of the vesical part of the urogenital sinus. The other layers of its wall develop from adjacent mesodermal tissue. The distal portions of the mesonephric ducts are incorporated into the trigone of the bladder.

38. **(E)** The femoral triangle contains the femoral nerve, artery, and vein, respectively, from lateral to medial. The femoral vein provides rapid access for volume expansion by large-bore IV catheter in the case of severe hypovolemia from trauma. The sartorius, inguinal ligament, and adductor longus border the femoral triangle.

39. **(C)** The patient is presenting with classic features of an acute arterial embolism: pallor, pain, paresthesias, and pulselessness. This is an acute emergency, and an angiogram followed by an embolectomy should be performed expeditiously. Venous ultrasound has no role in this situation as the clinical diagnosis is highly suggestive of an arterial embolism and not a venous thrombosis. Vasodilators may help improve collateral circulation and may be important as adjunctive therapy. Heparinization can help stabilize and prevent propagation of the clot. Fasciotomy would be useful if a compartment syndrome were suggested. In our patient, the likely source of the arterial embolism is cardiac, probably due to her atrial fibrillation.

40. **(C)** Depo-Provera is an extremely effective method of contraception when used appropriately with less than a 0.3% failure rate in the first year of use. However, unpredictable return of fertility after discontinuation as well as irregular bleeding and lack of protection against STDs may make other methods more attractive to many patients.

41. **(C)** In this setting, the possibility of heparin-induced thrombocytopenia (HIT) must be considered. There are two types. Type 1 is non–immune mediated and is rarely associated with a platelet level less than 100,000. This may occur in up to 30% of patients receiving heparin and is rarely associated with any complications. Type 2 is immune mediated and is also referred to as *white clot syndrome.* The thrombocytopenia is more severe and is associated with thromboembolic complications more so than hemorrhagic complications. Thromboembolism can occur in both venous and arterial systems and manifest clinically as pulmonary embolisms, strokes, limb ischemia, myocardial infarction, DVT, and so forth. Because of these serious complications, a high level of suspicion must be maintained, and if suspected, heparin must be discontinued. Heparin-dependent platelet antibodies may be helpful in confirming the diagnosis but are poorly sensitive. Alternative agents, such as lepirudin and danaparoid, must be considered or, in this case, even an inferior vena caval filter.

42. **(A)** Hair loss and weight gain are common complaints of women as they enter menopause but do not seem to be affected in a positive or negative way by hormone replacement. Unopposed estrogen therapy has been shown to be associated with an increased risk of endometrial cancer. The addi-

tion of appropriate amounts of progesterone reduces the risk of endometrial cancer to baseline. Vasomotor symptoms or "hot flashes" are very effectively treated by HRT.

43. **(E)** There is a noticeable discrepancy between the oxygen saturation and the oxygen tension (Pa_{O_2}). In this situation, a mutiple-wavelength co-oximeter should be run on the blood gas to ensure that there is no significant degree of alternative forms of hemoglobin. The co-oximeter uses four different wavelengths to determine the presence of alternative hemoglobin forms. They typically detect oxyhemoglobin, deoxyhemoglobin, carboxyhemoglobin, and methemoglobin. The clinical situation with the use of local anesthetics suggests methemoglobinemia. The blood gas is compatible with an arterial sample and is unlikely to be of venous origin. A pulmonary embolism may cause a respiratory alkalosis, as in this patient's ABGs, but the Pa_{O_2} would have been expected to be lower with a larger alveolar to arterial oxygen gradient. An intrapulmonary or an intracardiac shunt may produce hypoxemia that may not correct with oxygen administration. Orthodeoxia might also suggest a shunt process in a dependent area of the lung as seen with pulmonary arteriovenous malformations.

44. **(B)** Methemoglobin refers to the ferric state (Fe^{3+}) of iron in the heme moiety of hemoglobin. There is a low level of oxidation of ferrous iron (Fe^{2+}) to ferric iron in normal individuals, accounting for approximately 1% of the total hemoglobin. Most cases are acquired, but hereditary methemoglobinemia is also seen, most commonly related to a cytochrome b5 reductase deficiency (diaphorase or methemoglobin reductase) and hemoglobin M. Acquired cases are seen with use of or exposure to exogenous agents such as local anesthetics (benzocaine, lidocaine), nitrates, nitrites, chloroquine, dapsone, nitroglycerin, nitroprusside, and sulfonamides. Treatment for nonhereditary causes includes supportive care as well as the removal of any inciting oxidizing agent. The primary anti-

dote used is methylene blue (1–2 mg/kg IV), which accelerates the reduction of methemoglobin via NADPH (nicotinamide-adenine dinucleotide) methemoglobin reductase. At higher doses, methylene blue itself may cause methemoglobinemia. Clinically, cyanosis may be apparent with 10% to 15% methemoglobinemia, and symptoms occur at 20%. Its presence is commonly suggested by the presence of normal arterial tension (Pa_{O_2}) in the setting of low saturations. Because methemoglobin absorbs light at the same wavelength as oxy- and deoxyhemoglobin, pulse oximetry will tend to approach 85% regardless of the degree of methemoglobinemia. Therefore, it may either overestimate the degree of desaturation (when Sa_{O_2} is > 85%) or underestimate the desturation (when Sa_{O_2} is < 85%). Multiple-wavelength co-oximeter can be used to identify specifically the presence of methemoglobinemia.

45. **(B)** The ferric iron of methemoglobin is unable to bind oxygen, but the affinity of the other heme moieties within the same hemoglobin molecule increases. Therefore, oxygen is bound more tightly and delivered to the tissues less effectively. This is reflected by a left shift of the oxygen–hemoglobin dissociation curve and an "effective anemia."

46. **(B)** Type I primary collagen of postfetal skin; type II cartilage; type III primary collagen of fetal skin; type IV basement membrane (basal lamina); type V basement membrane (anchoring fibrils).

47. **(B)** Tuberous sclerosis is an inherited neurocutaneous disorder with several cutaneous manifestations, including fibromas arising from the nail unit.

48. **(C)** The classic triad of tuberous sclerosis consists of seizures, mental retardation, and adenoma sebaceum. White "ash leaf" macules are diagnostically important because they are usually present at birth.

49. **(D)** Pheochromocytomas are not part of the symptom complex associated with MEN 1

but are associated with MEN 2. Patients with MEN 1 have a genetic predisposition to the development of pituitary adenomas, hyperparathyroidism, and pancreatic islet cell tumors. An elevated serum parathyroid hormone (PTH) and elevation in serum calcium are sensitive markers for the diagnosis of this disease.

50. **(D)** The Blalock-Taussig procedure is performed in infants and young children born with cyanotic congenital heart disease. This surgery involves creation of a detour or shunt from the aorta to the pulmonary artery. The Blalock-Taussig procedure will relieve immediate signs and symptoms of the underlying heart defect but does not correct the heart defect. Additional surgeries may be necessary in the future to repair the defect itself.